SOFT TISSUE SARCOMAS

T0320694

Cancer Treatment and Research

WILLIAM L. MCGUIRE, *series editor*

R.B. Livingston, ed., Lung Cancer 1. 1981. ISBN 90-247-2393-9.

G.B. Humphrey, L.P. Dehner, G.B. Grindey and R.T. Acton, eds., Pediatric Oncology 1. 1981. ISBN 90-247-2408-2.

J.J. DeCosse and P. Sherlock, eds., Gastrointestinal Cancer 1. 1981. ISBN 90-247-2461-9.

J.M. Bennett, ed., Lymphomas 1, including Hodgkin's Disease. 1981. ISBN 90-247-2479-1.

C.D. Bloomfield, ed., Adult Leukemias 1. 1982. ISBN 90-247-2478-3.

D.F. Paulson, ed., Genitourinary Cancer 1. 1982. ISBN 90-247-2480-5.

F.M. Muggia, ed., Cancer Chemotherapy 1. 1983. ISBN 90-247-2713-8

G.B. Humphrey and G.B. Grindey, eds., Pancreatic Tumors in Children. ISBN 90-247-2702-2.

J.J. Costanzi, ed., Malignant Melanoma 1. 1983. ISBN 90-247-2706-5.

C.T. Griffiths and A.F. Fuller, eds., Gynecologic Oncology. 1983. ISBN 0-89838-555-5.

F.A. Greco, ed., Biology and Management of Lung Cancer. 1983. ISBN 0-89838-554-5.

M.D. Walker, ed., Oncology of the Nervous System. 1983. ISBN 0-89838-567-9.

D.J. Higby, Supportive Care in Cancer therapy. 1983. ISBN 0-89838-569-5.

R.B. Herberman, ed., Basic and Clinical Tumor Immunology. 1983. ISBN 0-89838-579-2.

J.M. Bennett, ed., Controversies in the Management of Lymphomas, including Hodgkin's Disease. 1983. ISBN 0-89838-586-5.

Soft Tissue Sarcomas

Edited by

LAURENCE H. BAKER

Division of Oncology
Wayne State University School of Medicine
Detroit, Michigan, U.S.A.

1983 **MARTINUS NIJHOFF PUBLISHERS**
a member of the KLUWER ACADEMIC PUBLISHERS GROUP
BOSTON / THE HAGUE / DORDRECHT / LANCASTER

Distributors

for the United States and Canada: Kluwer Boston, Inc., 190 Old Derby Street, Hingham, MA 02043, USA
for all other countries: Kluwer Academic Publishers Group, Distribution Center, P.O.Box 322, 3300 AH Dordrecht, The Netherlands

Library of Congress Cataloging in Publication Data

```
Library of Congress Cataloging in Publication Data
Main entry under title:

Soft tissue sarcomas.

   (Cancer treatment and research ; v. 15)
   Includes index.
   1. Sarcoma--Treatment--Addresses, essays, lectures.
I. Baker, Laurence H.  II. Series.  [DNLM: 1. Sarcoma.
2. Soft tissue neoplasms.  W1 CA693 v. 15 / WD 375 S681]
RC270.8.S63  1983     616.99'4          83-8138
ISBN 0-89838-584-9
```

ISBN 0-89838-584-9

PRINTED IN THE NETHERLANDS

Contents

Cancer Treatment and Research

Foreword

Where do you begin to look for a recent, authoritative article on the diagnosis or management of a particular malignancy? The few general oncology textbooks are generally out of date. Single papers in specialized journals are informative but seldom comprehensive; these are more often preliminary reports on a very limited number of patients. Certain general journals frequently publish good indepth reviews of cancer topics, and published symposium lectures are often the best overviews available. Unfortunately, these reviews and supplements appear sporadically, and the reader can never be sure when a topic of special interest will be covered.

Cancer treatment and Research is a series of authoritative volumes which aim to meet this need. It is an attempt to establish a critical mass of oncology literature covering virtually all oncology topics, revised frequently to keep the coverage up to date, easily available on a single library shelf or by a single personal subscription.

We have approached the problem in the following fashion. First, by dividing the oncology literature into specific subdivisions such as lung cancer, genitourinary cancer, pediatric oncology, etc. Second, by asking eminent authorities in each of these areas to edit a volume on the specific topic on an annual or biannual basis. Each topic and tumor type is covered in a volume appearing frequently and predictably, discussing current diagnosis, staging, markers, all forms of treatment modalities, basic biology, and more.

In Cancer Treatment and Research, we have an outstanding group of editors, each having made a major commitment to bring to this new series the very best literature in his or her field. Martinus Nijhoff Publishers has made an equally major commitment to the rapid publication of high quality books, and worldwide distribution.

Where can you go to find quickly a recent authoritative article on any major oncology problem? We hope that Cancer Treatment and Research provides an answer.

WILLIAM L. McGUIRE
Series Editor

Preface

While the soft tissue sarcomas comprise only 0.7% of all cancers, nonetheless they represent a major challenge to the biomedical research effort. Thus far the major successes in oncology today have occurred in malignancies of hematopoietic origin. The common epithelial cancers remain a major health problem. Sarcomas are unique in that they may serve as a model for the successful combination of therapeutic strategies in the more common epithelial malignancies. The cell of origin of the majority of soft tissue sarcomas arises from mesenchymal tissue, as do the hematopoietic malignancies, and unlike the epithelial cancer. Yet, unlike the hematopoietic malignancies, most soft tissue sarcomas begin as a tumor mass in a distant anatomic site and like many epithelial tumors, present the therapeutic problem of achieving local control.

This book is intended to provide a current review of the clinical activities of the major disciplines involved in the management of patients with soft tissue sarcomas. Whenever appropriate, emphasis will be given to combined modality approaches.

Pathology
The exact criteria for establishing the histologic cell of origin and for establishing the grade of individual sarcomas has not been consistent among pathologists. Disagreement in diagnosis and grading is frequent. In addition new diagnoses (malignant fibrous histiocytoma) have been popularized in recent years that were not in common usage previously. These differences and changes has served to complicate comparison of current clinical trials with previously reported results. Electron microscopy is gaining acceptance in helping to define some of these issues. Another aid has been the establishment of pathology review panels, particularly in studies involving multiple institutions and disciplines.

Diagnostic Strategy
A proposed diagnostic strategy for the evaluation of soft tissue sarcomas is offered. The strategy is based on the anatomic behavior and includes the medical history, a physical examination, scintigraphic, conventional and com-

puted imaging, and biopsy. The rational application of these tests in an orderly fashion will yield a most effective and complete preoperative characterization of the sarcoma and its local and distant extent.

Staging
It is important to stage malignant neoplasms in order to: (1) plan effective therapy, (2) make accurate prognostications and, (3) compare similar lesions and various methods of treatment in end-result studies. No uniformly accepted staging system for sarcomas exists. Three staging systems are presented and analyzed. Clearly more work is needed in this area.

Surgical Treatment
Surgical ablation remains the predominant method of choice in dealing with sarcomas. Several investigational techniques are discussed. Precise surgical procedures are described for the various anatomical locations. For best results, the definitive surgical procedure should be planned if possible at the time of surgery. The surgeon's aim in the treatment of soft tissue sarcoma is the complete irradiation of the sarcoma while at the same time preserving maximum function.

Special surgical considerations include: (1) the primary excision of a retroperitoneal sarcoma, (2) the excision of a metastatic tumor as part of cyto reduction, and (3) the palliative excision of metastatic tumor in patients in order to enhance comfort and assist further palliative therapy.

Radiotherapy
While there is little enthusiasm for the treatment of localized soft tissue sarcomas by curative radiation therapy alone there is increasing interest in exploring the role of this form of therapy as an adjuvant to surgery (either pre-operatively or post-operatively) and with the use of chemotherapy as an adjuvant to radiotherapy alone or combined with surgery. Radiation therapy appears to play a significant role in advancing the concept of limb-salvage procedures for extremity lesions. For small and moderate sized lesions the combinations of limited surgery and post-operative radiation therapy has achieved the same absolute 5-year disease free survival rate as radical surgery while maintaining a functional extremity in 85% of patients.

Chemotherapy
The chemotherapy of soft tissue sarcomas is primarily based upon adriamycin. In 1972 the role of adriamycin was established to produce a moderate frequency of clinical responses. Several thousands of patients have been entered into clinical trials in an effort to establish and improve the chemotherapeutic management of this set of diseases. Multiple combinations have been explored based

in part upon the premise of therapeutic synergism for adriamycin when combined with either DTIC or cyclophosphamide in experimental murine models. Extensive efforts have been launched to alter the route and schedule of adriamycin so as to improve the efficacy and reduce the toxicity of this drug. Since the mechanism of death of these patients is primarily dictated by hematogenous metastases, these efforts with chemotherapy seem warranted.

As a result of these efforts the optimism the clinicians can enjoy when approaching the patient with a soft tissue sarcoma is increasing. Nonetheless therapeutic results are still far from satisfactory and justify continual and indeed enhanced efforts are directed at improved modalities of treatment.

Perfusion Chemotherapy
Limb perfusion is an interesting technique that presents some theoretical advantages for delivery of high concentrations of drug to the tumor bed; however, it also presents some major logistic and practical problems. Eilber reports a local disease control rate of over 98% in a sequential series of 110 patients with extremity soft tissue sarcomas treated by intraarterial adriamycin, radiation therapy and surgical excision.

Infusion Chemotherapy
By utilizing a continuous infusion of adriamycin, Benjamin and co-workers have demonstrated that substantially higher adriamycin doses may be given than by the standard intermittent single dose rapid infusion schedule. Not only can the cumulative dose of adriamycin be almost doubled but the resultant cardiac dose as assessed by endomyocardial biopsy is less. In incorporating this dose schedule of adriamycin into a combination chemotherapy program with planned surgical debulking the median survival of a series of 50 consecutive patients was 21 months in comparison to approximately 9–12 months in other large series.

Adjuvant Chemotherapy Disease
A key question regarding the management of soft tissue sarcomas is whether or not chemotherapy is a useful adjuvant. To prove the value of chemotherapy is a most difficult task considering all the complexities of this group of diseases. Rosenberg et al. at the National Cancer Institute report a positive therapeutic trial. This random prospective trial suggests that chemotherapy is of benefit in prolonging disease free and overall survival in patients with soft tissue sarcomas of the extremities. Other studies using historical controls are cited in support of the conclusion that chemotherapy is recommended as an adjuvant.

List of Contributors

BAKER, L.H., Department of Internal Medicine, Division of Oncology, Wayne State University, University Health Center 7C, 4201 St. Antoine, Detroit, MI 48201, U.S.A.

BENJAMIN, R.S., The University of Texas System Cancer Center, M.D. Anderson Hospital and Tumor Institute, Department of Internal Medicine, Section of Melanoma/Sarcoma, 6723 Bertner Drive, Houston, TX 77030, U.S.A.

EILBER, F.R., Division of Oncology, University of California, Los Angeles, School of Medicine, The Center for the Health Sciences, Los Angeles, CA 90024, U.S.A.

KERNS, L.L., The University of Chicago, Department of Surgery, Section of Orthopedics, Box 102, 950 East 59th Street, Chicago, IL 60637, U.S.A.

LEDGERWOOD, A., Department of Surgery, Wayne State University, 540 E. Canfield, Detroit, MI 48201, U.S.A.

LINDBERG, R.D., The University of Texas, M.D. Anderson Hospital and Tumor Institute at Houston, 6723 Bertner Avenue, Houston, TX 77030, U.S.A.

LUCAS, C.E., Department of Surgery, Wayne State University, 540 E. Canfield, Detroit, MI 48201, U.S.A.

ROSENBERG, S.A., National Cancer Institute, Building 10, Room 10–116, Bethesda, MD 20205, U.S.A.

RYAN, J.R., Department of Orthopedics, Wayne State University, University Health Center 7C, 4201 St. Antoine, Detroit, MI 48201, U.S.A.

SAMSON, M.K., Department of Internal Medicine, Division of Oncology, Wayne State University, University Health Center 7C, 4201 St. Antoine, Detroit, MI 48201, U.S.A.

SIMON, M.A., The University of Chicago, Department of Surgery, Section of Orthopedics, Box 102, 950 East 59th Street, Chicago, IL 60637, U.S.A.

TANG, C.-K., Department of Pathology, University of Maryland, School of Medicine, 22 South Greene Street, Baltimore, MD 21201, U.S.A.

YAP, B.-S., The University of Texas System Cancer Center, M.D. Anderson Hospital and Tumor Institute, Department of Internal Medicine, Section of Melanoma/Sarcoma, 6723 Bertner Drive, Houston, TX 77030, U.S.A.

1. Changing Concepts in Pathology

CHIK-KWUN TANG

Over the past two decades or so, several major developments have brought our knowledge of soft tissue sarcomas to the current state. The introduction of the histogenetic concept of a group of sarcomas, the malignant fibrous histiocytomas (MFH), has resulted in an extension of the classification and a decrease in the diagnosis of pleomorphic liposarcomas, pleomorphic rhabdomyosarcomas, and unclassifiable or undifferentiated sarcomas. Though the cell of origin is still a debatable issue, MFH has been accepted as a distinct clinicopathologic entity. With the aid of electron microscopy (EM), pathologists have been able to observe the cytologic details which cannot be seen by light microscopy (LM), thus extending the spectrum of morphology. Some of these ultrastructure structures have confirmed the histogenetic concepts derived from LM such as those of rhabdomyosarcomas, leiomyosarcomas, etc., but some other EM findings have created new arguments on previously favored concepts, e.g., melanin pigments in clear cell sarcomas creating doubt on their synovial origin, etc. Nonetheless, many of the EM structures have been proven helpful in subclassifying sarcomas. Careful epidemiologic observations have linked, for instance, polyvinyl chloride (PVC) to angiosarcomas of liver. Retrospective, clinicopathologic studies have also proved to be an important approach, without which, the concept of alveolar soft part sarcoma would not have been borne.

Factors Probably Responsible for the Development of Sarcomas

From various investigations, there are apparently more than one factor responsible for the development of sarcomas. Ever since Rous' discovery [1, 2], virus has always been a suspect as a causative agent of sarcomas. Under the electron microscope the viral particles were found to be spherical, measuring 70–80 mu, limited by a smooth external membrane having very electron dense cores and attached to the plasma membranes and not in the cytoplasm of the Rous sarcoma cells [3]. In a human liposarcoma, virus-like particles were found but were morphologically different from Rous sarcoma viruses [4]. Ultrastructural

Baker, L.H. (ed.), Soft Tissue Sarcomas. ISBN 0-89838-584-9
© *1983 Martinus Nijhoff Publishers, Boston/The Hague/Dordrecht/Lancaster. Printed in the Netherlands.*

evidence of viral particles has so far not been observed in the sarcomas studied by us.

Immunologic and cytotoxicity studies [5, 6] have shown that different types of sarcomas shared a common antigen. However, this antigen could not be related to antigens of known human viruses [5].

Irradiation is a well known factor in cases of sarcomas arising at the sites of previous irradiation therapy for other cancers, the so-called post-irradiation sarcomas. Various post-irradiation sarcomas have been observed, including malignant fibrous histiocytomas, fibrosarcomas, desmoid tumors, synovial (tenosynovial) sarcomas, myosarcomas, angiosarcomas, neurogenic sarcomas and undifferentiated sarcomas [7–9]. Post-irradiation sarcomas are rare but the exact rate of occurrence is difficult to determine.

Vinyl chloride, thorotrast and arsenic are known to be able to induce angiosarcomas (Kupffer cell sarcomas) of the liver [10]. In patients who were not known to have been exposed to any of these chemicals, chemicals structurally similar to vinyl chloride such as chloroprene, styrene and trichloroethylene might be responsible for the development of their hepatic angiosarcomas [11]. Considering that endothelium and Kupffer cells are basically the same type of cells, one would wonder whether these chemicals may also be responsible for the development of some angiosarcomas of the skin and soft tissue. Extravasated thorotrast was reported to have resulted in spindle cell sarcomas at the site of injection [12].

Host factors probably also play a role under certain circumstances. For instance, immune deficiency likely predisposes patients to Kaposi's sarcoma [13]. In patients with von Recklinhausen's disease (neurofibromatosis) there is a strong possibility that the occurrence of various malignant tumors, including sarcomas, reflects expression of abnormal genomes in various tissues [14].

Histogenesis and Classification

Soft tissues are neither an organ nor a precise histologic term, which makes it almost impossible to define soft tissue sarcomas. Stout and Lattes included all non-epithelial tissues that are outside the bones in the soft tissue category, excluding bone marrow and lymph nodes [15]. Tumors that arise from these soft tissues can, therefore, be designated as soft tissue sarcomas or mesenchymal sarcomas. Based on the cell of origin, most malignant soft tissue tumors would fall into the categories of fibrohistiocytic, fibrous, adipose tissue, muscular, synovial, vascular and peripheral nerve sarcomas. There remains a small group of rare sarcomas of uncertain origins, which are usually designated with descriptive terms, e.g., clear cell sarcomas, alveolar soft part sarcoma, etc. Readers who are interested in the historic review of classification of soft tissue tumors are referred to ref. 8.

Traditionally, the type of a given sarcoma is based primarily on its histologic and cytologic similarity to the tissue where the tumor occurs. For instance, a rhabdomyosarcoma is considered a sarcoma of the skeletal muscle cells. The exact cell or origin actually is not as clear as the term indicates, in that whether it arises directly from myoblasts or from the multipotential primitive mesenchymal cells (cells that can differentiate into myoblasts, fibroblasts, etc.) [16]. At present, there seems to be no clear answer to this question. If sarcomas are derived from multipotential primitive mesenchymal cells, it would be entirely possible that, because of their multipotentiality, different derivatives, e.g., myoblasts, fibroblasts, etc., may be present within any given sarcoma, with predominance of one of the derivatives. In an ultrastructural study, malignant fibrous histiocytomas, pleomorphic liposarcomas and rhabdomyosarcomas were found to share certain morphologic features which are considered to be sufficient to support the concept of a common histogenesis for tumors of mesenchymal origin [17]. That the possibility of a primitive mesenchymal origin is probably true with sarcomas that have been observed to be composed of several types of cells, e.g., malignant fibrous histiocytomas [18]. For many other sarcomas, the original cells may have

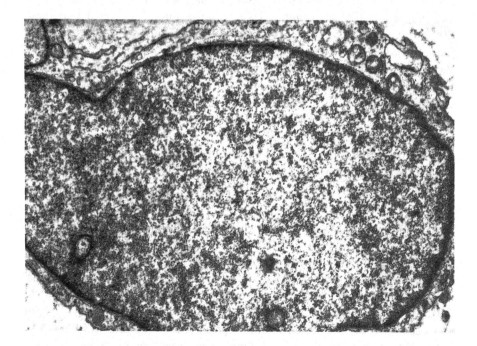

Fig. 1. An undifferentiated mesenchymal cell in a liposarcoma characterized by scanty cytoplasmic organelles, including rough endoplasmic reticulum (RER), mitochondria, lysosomal granules and a few fine filaments (EM).

been the genetically determined precursor cells with the potential to differentiate into a specific cell type during a neoplastic process but phenotypically cannot yet be recognized as precursor cells specific for that cell type. In well differentiated leiomyosarcomas, features characterizing smooth muscle cells are easily found in the majority of tumor cells [19, 20 and author's own cases]. In this particular instance, it would be inconceivable that multipotential mesenchymal cells are the cells of origin of the well-differentiated leiomyosarcomas with a relatively uniform cellular population. Figure 1 illustrates an undifferentiated mesenchymal cell by EM.

The Changing Concepts in Individual Sarcomas

1. Fibrohistiocytic and fibrocytic sarcomas

Malignant fibrous histiocytoma (malignant fibrous xanthoma or fibroxanthosarcoma): The identification of this group of sarcomas in the early 60's was the result of the belief that fibrous xanthoma is not always benign [21]. After reviewing more than a thousand cases, it was found that 1% of the tumors behaved in a malignant fashion. Tissue culture studies suggested that these tumors originate from tissue histiocytes which function as 'facultative fibroblasts' [22]. These clinicopathologic and tissue culture studies formed the basis of the current terminology, malignant fibrous histiocytoma (MFH). Though MFH represents a part of the spectrum of benign and malignant soft tissue tumors considered to be histiocytic origin, it has been accepted as a distinct clinicopathologic entity [23–25]. MFH usually occurs in patients between 50 and 70 years of age, more often in deep than superficial tissues, and mostly in the extremities but also in trunks, abdominal and retroperitoneal cavities [24, 25].

Grossly, MFHs are well-circumscribed but non-encapsulated, white or tannish, firm tumors (Fig. 2) and usually measure 5 cm or larger. Before being recognized as an entity, MFHs were diagnosed as either pleomorphic rhabdomyosarcomas or pleomorphic liposarcomas for an obvious reason that all three types often acquire pleomorphic features with spindle, round and giant cells. The majority of MFHs show storiform and/or fascicular patterns and pleomorphic cellular features (Fig. 3A). Most of the tumor cells are spindle, resembling fibroblasts or irregularly round, mimicking histiocytes (Figs. 3A, 3B). The resemblance is also observed at the EM level (Figs. 4A, 4B). Tumor giant cells and less frequently, Touton-type giant cells and cells with abundant foamy cytoplasm are noted. Mitotic figures vary from tumor to tumor. Chronic inflammatory infiltrates may be present. These histologic and cytologic features, in combination, are highly characteristic of MFHs, but a single feature should not be regarded as an absolute criterion, such as storiform pattern, which may be

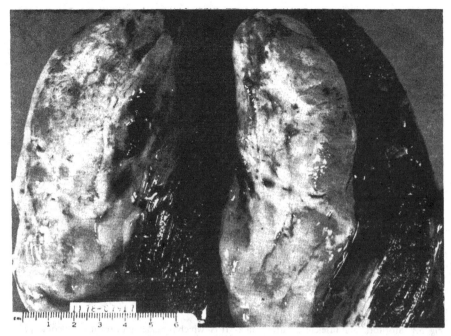

Fig. 2. Gross appearance of a MFH. Although infiltrating the skeletal muscle, the lobulated tumor is well-circumscribed. The tumor is firm and homogeneous for the most part, but fibrous areas (lighter areas) are also observed.

quite conspicuous, for instance in leiomyosarcomas. In addition to pleomorphism, the location of MFHs that they occur in the skeletal muscle [24, 25] may be responsible for the diagnostic difficulties in distinguishing them from pleomorphic rhabdomyosarcomas. If cross striations are found either by light microscopy (usually with PTAH stain) or EM, the latter diagnosis can be established. The distinction between MFH and liposarcoma may be difficult. If lipoblasts are present or mixed features of MFH and liposarcoma are observed within the same tumor, it is classified as pleomorphic liposarcoma [24].

In addition to the pleomorphic form, the morphologic spectrum of MFHs has been expanded to include myxoid [25, 26], inflammatory (acute inflammatory infiltrates) [23, 25, 27, 28] and angiomatoid MFHs [28]. The prognosis of the myxoid MFH was found to be better than that of the non-myxoid MFH [26]; that of the inflammatory variant, an aggressive and lethal lesion [27]. However, no difference in prognosis was observed among the subtypes of MFHs in another series [25]. Other parameters, such as size, location, etc., are important prognostic factors.

The results of tissue culture seemed to have ended the controversy, as pointed out by Ozzello *et al.*, regarding the nature of tumor cells and histogenesis of MFHs [22]. The morphology and the ameboid outgrowth, and the phagocytic

6

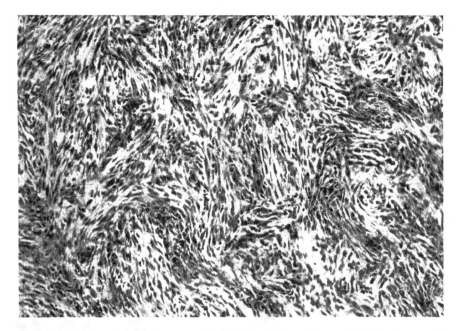

Fig. 3A. Storiform and fascicular patterns in a MFH, which is made up of relatively pleomorphic neoplastic spindle cells (LM).

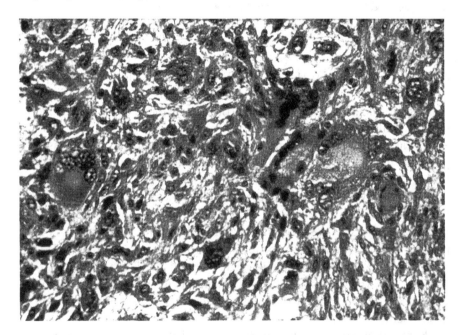

Fig. 3B. The pleomorphic patterns are more conspicuous in this MFH than those in A, with mixed spindle, oval and giant cells. The cells that possess abundant cytoplasm resemble histiocytes and the spindle cells are fibroblast-like cells. The background shows scanty collagen fibers (LM).

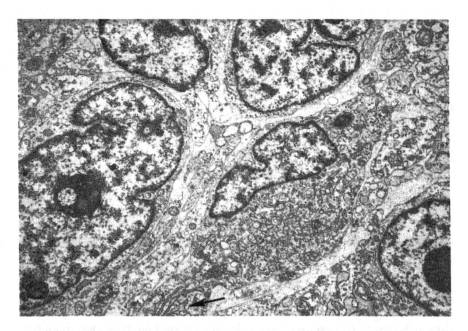

Fig. 4A. Both fibroblast-like and undifferentiated cells are present in this particular area of a MFH. The former show dilated RER in which finely granular material is present (arrow). The latter are similar to that in Figure 1 with only scanty cytoplasmic organelles (EM).

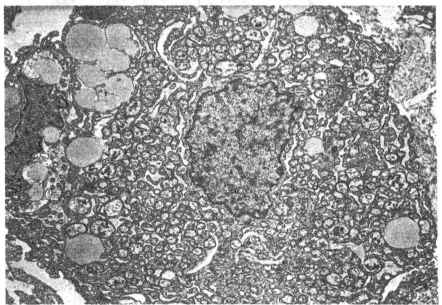

Fig. 4B. Histiocyte-like cell in MFH showing pseudopodia (arrow) (cytoplasmic process). The abundant mitochondria and prominent RER and the absence of lysosomes or phagosomes suggest a productive rather than phagocytic state (EM).

activities of tumor cells as observed in culture led to the belief of histiocytic origin of MFHs. Based on the observations that fibroblasts may morphologically be similar to histiocytes and show phagocytic activities, the difficulties in interpreting the differentiation of histiocytes into fibroblasts and that EM revealed several types of tumor cells, including undifferentiated cells, Fu *et al.* suggested that all types of cells observed in MFHs may derive from the same undifferentiated stem cells [18]. The histogenesis of MFH remains a controversial subject. The difficulty in drawing a conclusive answer is derived from the difficulty in defining histiocytes and fibroblasts [8]. Morphologic studies have suggested that dermatofibrosarcoma protuberans [29] and fibrosarcomas [30] are probably related to MFHs.

The clinicopathologic aspects of dermatofibrosarcoma and fibrosarcomas have been well defined [8]. From the diagnostic point of view, it may be worthwhile to point out that, despite the characteristic 'herring bone' appearance in fibrosarcomas (Fig. 5), the packed cellularity may also be a pattern seen in leiomyosarcomas.

It is interesting to observe the changing definition of desmoid tumors [8], another type of fibrous tumor. The author feels that the understanding of the clinical behavior of desmoid tumors is more important than the argument

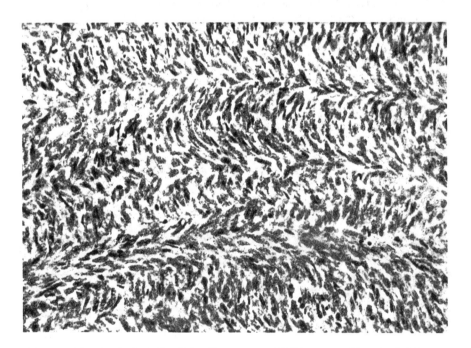

Fig. 5. Fascicles of packed spindle cells in a fibrosarcoma, which are arranged in such a fashion as to resemble herring bone. The sharp ends of the nuclei are also in favor of a fibrosarcoma, as opposed to the blunt ends of nuclei in leiomyosarcoma (LM).

whether it is a benign or malignant tumor. Despite its similarity to fibroma in terms of cytologic appearance, desmoid tumor is a locally aggressive but extremely rarely metastasizing fibrous tumor [8].

2. Sarcomas of adiposise tissue

These tumors can present with various gross and microscopic features as reflected by the numerous terms used by different investigators [8]. For practical purpose, liposarcomas can be divided into low and high grade subcategories, based essentially on cellularity. The differentiated or well-differentiated and myxoid (Figs. 6A, 6B, & inset) variants belong to the low grade group in view of their favorable outcome and extremely low incidence of metastasis. The high grade liposarcomas are cellular with conspicuous spindle cells (fibroblastic liposarcoma) (Fig. 7), mixed spindle and giant cells (pleomorphic liposarcoma) or round cells (lipoblastic liposarcoma) [8]. In the event that problems in differential diagnosis arise, identification of lipoblasts (Fig. 6B, inset) is helpful for establishing the diagnosis of a liposarcoma. Fully malignant liposarcomas may become better differentiated when they recur. Conversely, a well-differentiated liposarcoma may acquire such malignant features that its adipose nature may be obscured, which may be regarded as dedifferentiation. Spindle cell and pleomorphic lipomas (Fig. 8) may be mistaken for liposarcomas [31, 32].

3. Sarcomas of muscular origin

Rhabdomyosarcomas, sarcoma of the skeletal muscle that occur in adults, are predominantly the pleomorphic type, characterized by spindle, round, polygonal, strap-shaped, racquet-shaped or spider-web cells with abundant cytoplasm (Fig. 9A). Gross striations are present in some tumors (Fig. 9A, inset). Mitoses are numerous. The amount of collagen in the background varies. After the recognition of MHF, the incidence of pleomorphic rhabdomyosarcoma is expected to decline because diagnosis of many of the latter has been revised [24]. However, since EM may reveal Z-bands associated with myofilaments [17, 33] (Fig. 9B) (corresponding to cross striations on LM), pleomorphic rhabdomyosarcomas may not be as rare as Weiss and Enzinger indicated [24]. Recently, Hajdu introduced a term 'rhabdomyoblastoma' to designate a variant that is lethal and composed predominantly of round or polygonal tumor cells [8]. Grossly, rhabdomyosarcomas are fleshy, relatively soft and greyish (Fig. 9C). Areas of necrosis may be present.

Leiomyosarcomas have a widespread distribution [8, 34, 35]. Although rare outside the organs in which smooth muscle is a normal anatomic structure, e.g.,

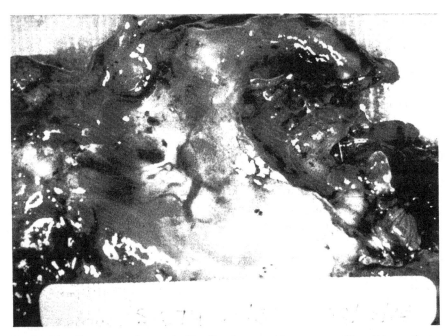

Fig. 6A. Myxoliposarcoma characterized by glistening, myxoid appearance of the soft tumor tissue. Areas of hemorrhage are apparent.

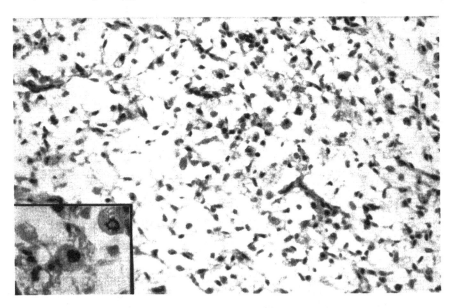

Fig. 6B. Microscopic appearance of a myxoliposarcoma from a different case. The background is identical to that of a myxoma of soft tissue. Compressed capillaries are present. The tumor cells are either spindle or round with few mitoses (inset). Many round cells display vacuoles and vesicles in the cytoplasm, pushing the nuclei to the periphery (inset), all of which are features of lipoblasts (LM).

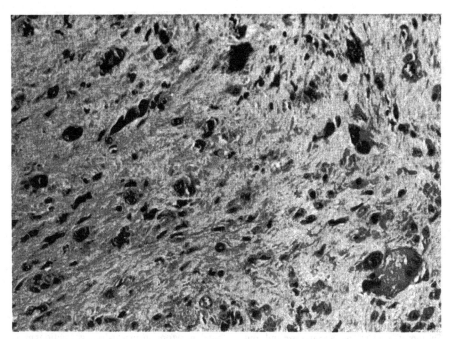

Fig. 7. Pleomorphic liposarcoma showing an area that may be interpreted as MFH or rhabdomyosarcoma, but other parts of the tumor are typical of a liposarcoma (not shown in this microphotograph) (LM).

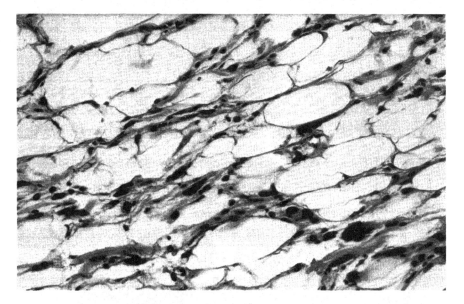

Fig. 8. A pleomorphic lipoma removed from the neck. The degree of atypia and pleomorphism of tumor cells makes the distinction from a low grade (well-differentiated) liposarcoma difficult. The location, the well-circumscribed margin of the tumor should all be taken into consideration (LM).

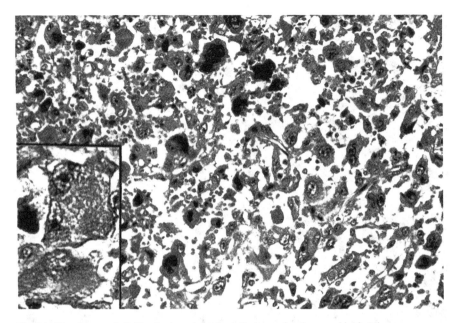

Fig. 9A. The characteristic histologic and cytologic features of a pleomorphic rhabdomyosarcoma. The tumor cells vary in shape and size and contain abundant cytoplasm in which cross striations may be found (inset – PTAH stain). The pleomorphism of the nuclei is even greater, ranging from round to extremely irregular and hyperchromatic and from single nuclear to multinuclear. The nucleoli are so prominent that an interpretation of Reed-Sternberg cell may result (LM).

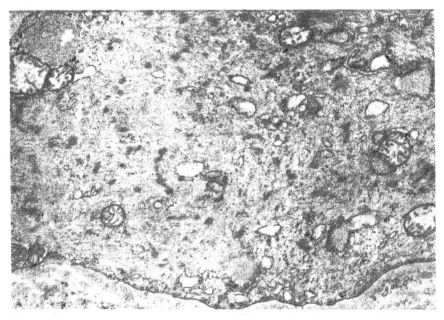

Fig. 9B. EM of the biopsy material from the same tumor reveals banded filaments (EM).

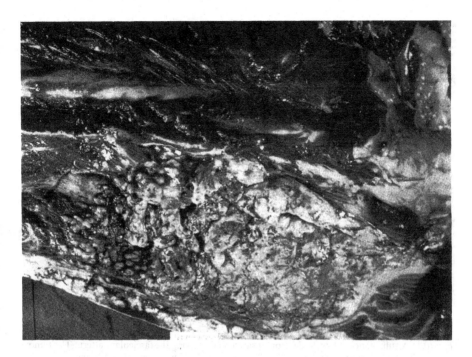

Fig. 9C. The gross appearance of a rhabdomyosarcoma from another case. The tumor tissue is grey and soft to relatively firm. Multiple satellite tumor nodules are observed in the adjacent skeletal muscle.

gastrointestinal tract, uterus, etc., leiomyosarcomas can occur anywhere blood vessels with smooth muscle walls are present. Low grade leiomyosarcomas closely resemble normal smooth muscle cells with few mitoses (Fig. 10A). As the tumors become less differentiated, the cellularity and mitoses increase. The tumor cells may acquire an epithelioid feature (Fig. 10B). By electron microscopy, the most characteristic features are the myofilaments associated with dense bodies (Fig. 10C). Other EM structures include dense plagues, pinocytotic vesicles and basal lamina. In general, the better the differentiation the tumor is, the more conspicuous these EM structures are.

4. Synovial (tendosynovial) sarcomas

The concept that sarcomas can arise from synovial tissue has been well accepted. Though the synovial nature of the biphasic variant (composed of both glandular epithelium and spindle cells) is undoubted, that of the monophasic variant (Figs. 11A, 11B) remains a controversy [36]. The location of tumors [36, 37], the EM resemblance to synovial tissue [36] and the similar characteristics to synovium on

14

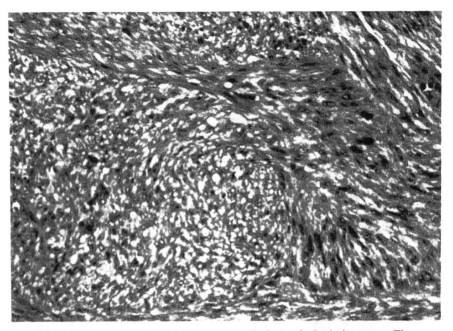

Fig. 10A. A subcutaneous low grade leiomyosarcoma displaying the fascicular pattern. The tumor cells possess relatively abundant cytoplasm, as compared to cells of fibrosarcoma. The nuclei are relatively pleomorphic and atypical and mitoses are few (LM).

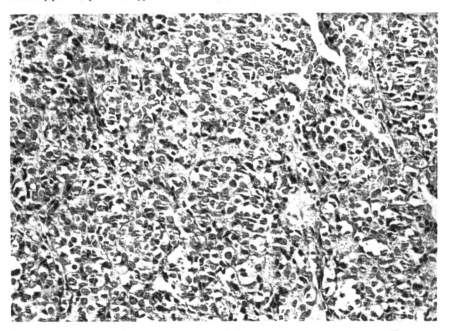

Fig. 10B. A more cellular leiomyosarcoma with prominent epithelioid cells with vacuolated cytoplasm (LM).

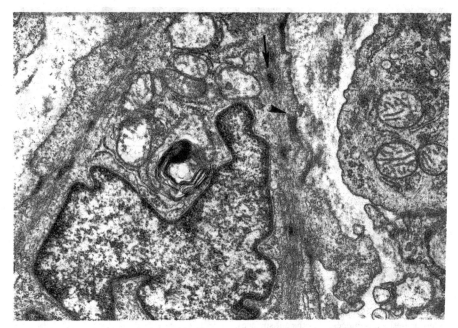

Fig. 10C. A tumor cell from a leiomyosarcoma showing pinocytotic vesicles and dense plaques (arrowhead) along the plasma membrane and myofilaments associated with dense bodies (arrow) in the cytoplasm, features that are characteristic of smooth muscle cells. Interrupted basal lamina is also present (EM).

culture [38] appear to support the existence of a monophasic synovial sarcoma. The monophasic variants behave more aggressively than their biphasic counterparts [36] (Fig. 11C).

5. Sarcomas of vascular origin

Angiosarcomas (Fig. 12) occur in skin, superficial and deep soft tissues [39], and other organs, e.g., liver [10] and uterus and ovary [40], etc. The term, angiosarcoma, is preferred over hemangiosarcoma or lymphangiosarcoma because they may histologically be indistinguishable from each other. According to Hajdu [8], the term lymphangiosarcoma began to appear in the literature after Stewart and Treve's report of post-mastectomy angiosarcoma in 1948 [41]. Pre-existing lymphedema was found in the site of lymphangiosarcoma in 40 out of 44 patients [42]. Weibel-Palade bodies, specific EM structures for endothelial cells, are rare in angiosarcoma cells, but other EM features, e.g., lumen formation and duplicate basal lamina, are consistent with endothelial in nature [14, 43].

Like angiosarcomas, Kaposi's sarcomas are of endothelial origin [44], but

16

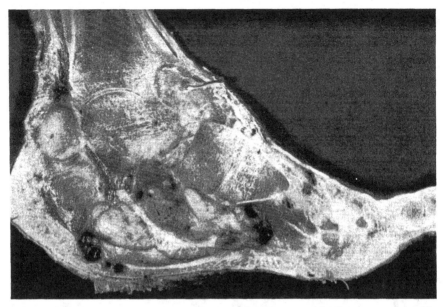

Fig. 11A. Synovial sarcoma involving fascia, muscle joints, bones and subcutaneous tissue. The tumor is fleshy and bulges from the cut surfaces.

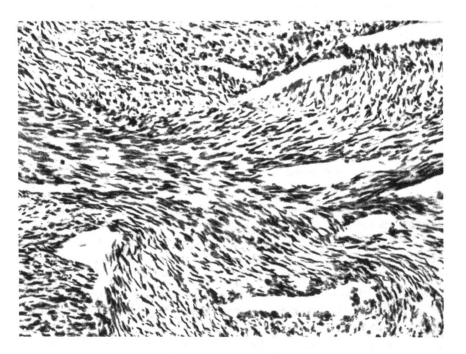

Fig. 11B. Microscopic features of the same tumor with packed spindle cells in which clear spaces and slits are observed, characteristic of a monophasic synovial sarcoma (LM).

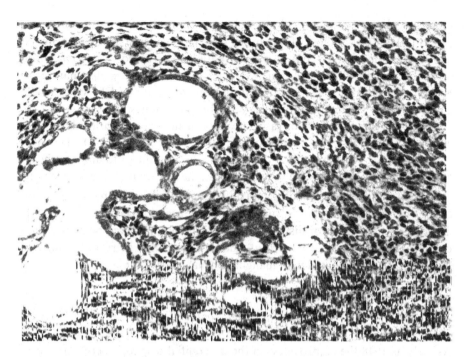

Fig. 11C. A biphasic synovial sarcoma showing gland-like structures in the midst of spindle cells. Focal infiltration by lymphocytes is present. (ILM).

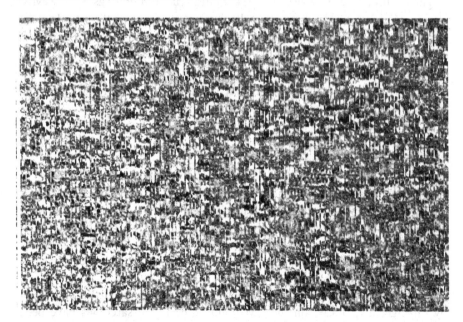

Fig. 12. Angiosarcoma showing a cellular area in which irregular slit-like spaces are barely visible, which are lined by hyperchromatic and pleomorphic tumor cells (ILM).

their clinical manifestation, pathologic features (Fig. 13) and behavior are completely different from those of the former [45]. The incidence of second primary malignant tumors is markedly increased in patients with Kaposi's sarcoma, most of which are lymphoreticular malignancies [46]. The endothelial nature of Kaposi's sarcoma has been confirmed by histochemical and EM studies [44], particularly the latter which revealed Weibel-Palade bodies.

Within the same category of vascular tumor, hemangiopericytoma is a histogenetically related but clinicopathologically distinct entity [47–50]. The high vascular pattern in other types of sarcomas makes it difficult to diagnose hemangiopericytoma [51]. Though variations exist, the EM studies have consistently shown basal lamina surrounding individual tumor cells and separating tumor cells from the endothelial cells, supporting the concept of pericytic nature [51]. The diagnostic criteria for distinguishing benign and malignant hemangiopericytomas are not clear cut but recent studies showed that increased cellularity and mitoses are associated with malignant behavior [49, 50].

6. Malignant Schwannoma (neurogenic sarcoma) (Fig. 14)

As early as 1948 the controversy on the differential diagnosis between neurogenic sarcoma and fibrosarcoma was apparent [52]. It is interesting that similar diagnostic problems still exist. The recent ultrastructural findings of long cytoplasmic processes surrounded by basal lamina, not only confirm the neural nature of malignant Schwannomas but also are useful in establishing the diagnosis when diagnostic difficulties arise [20, 53]. The fact that pleomorphic and atypical cells can be observed in some neurofibromas and Schwannomas, may make distinction between benign and malignant Schwannomas difficult. Mitoses, even rare, should raise the suspicion of the latter.

7. Miscellaneous sarcomas

Alveolar soft part sarcoma was first described as a distinct clinicopathologic entity by Christopherson et al. [54]. The histogenesis even with the aid of EM, is still debated between myogenic [55] and paraganglionic [56] origins. Despite the uncertain origin, the rhomboid inclusions found in tumor cells by EM are highly characteristic of alveolar soft part sarcoma and are thus helpful when there is a diagnostic problem.

The term, clear cell sarcoma (Fig. 15), was introduced to the medical literature by Enzinger [57]. Based on the EM findings, clear cell sarcomas have been interpreted as a form of synovial sarcoma [8, 58]. The findings of melanin pigments led to the conclusion that the reported case was an atypical melanoma

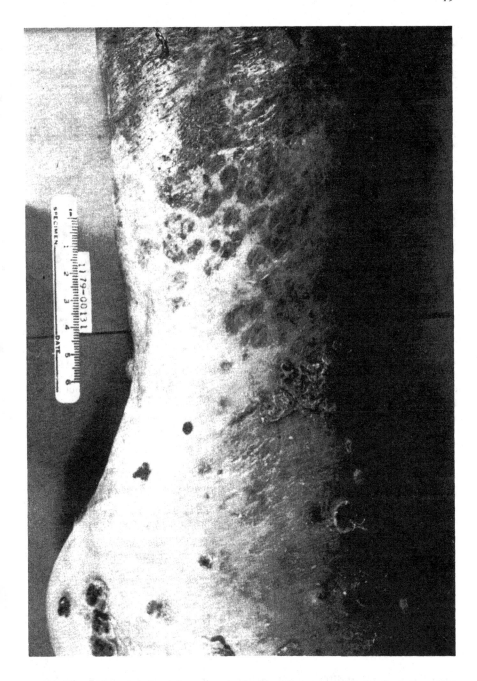

Fig. 13. The product of a below-knee amputation for Kaposi's sarcoma with characteristic, multifocal involvement and dark color. Some lesions appear ulcerated and are covered by grey necrotic debris.

20

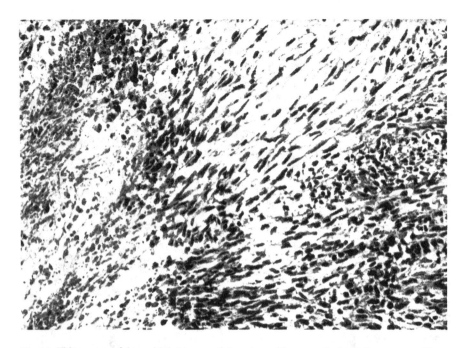

Fig. 14. This was one of the multiple tumor nodules removed from a patient with known neurofibromatosis. Histologically, this tumor is packed with spindle cells for the most part but less cellular areas are also present. The spindle cells may be difficult to distinguish from those of cellular leiomyosarcomas, or fibrosarcomas (it was diagnosed as such elsewhere), but the wavy appearance of the cytoplasmic processes is most compatible with malignant schwannoma. Necrosis is marked (LM).

and that the histogenesis of clear cell sarcomas may vary [59].

Epithelioid sarcoma is a term introduced in 1970 [60] to designate a rare form of sarcoma that shows necrosis, epithelioid and spindle cells, features that may be confused with other benign and malignant lesions, e.g., granuloma, metastatic carcinoma. Recent studies suggested that these sarcomas are synovial in origin [61]. Malignant granular cells tumors, extraskeletal Ewing's sarcoma, extraosseous osteogenic sarcoma, paraganglioma and teratoma may occur in soft tissue [8].

The Contributions of Special Techniques in Soft Tissue Sarcomas

Despite the fact that different mesenchymal derivatives may share certain histologic and cytologic features, light microscopy remains the most important method in the diagnosis of soft tissue sarcomas. It is expected that overlapping morphology might result in controversies in the classification. Special histo-

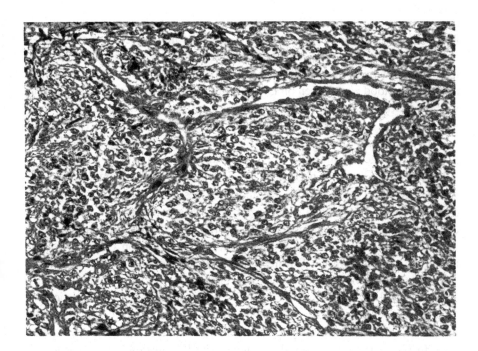

Fig. 15. A recurrent clear cell sarcoma displaying clear cytoplasm in tumor cells. The tumor was diagnosed as 'metastatic adenocarcinoma' on the first biopsy. Thorough clinical investigation revealed no tumor elsewhere (LM).

chemical stains, e.g., Masson trichrome, Phosphotungstic Acid Hematoxylin (PTAH), etc., have limited values. For instance, PTAH only occasionally demonstrates cross striations in rhabdomyosarcomas but the positive finding would make a definitive classification of a pleomorphic sarcoma. In view of the high resolution, EM has been used to demonstrate the characteristic structures that cannot be identified by light microscopy. After many years of cumulative efforts, virtually all types of sarcomas have been examined by EM [20]. Many of the EM features have been proven to be helpful in diagnosis. For this reason EM is no longer a pure experimental tool but a tool for practical use as well.

Like any special tool, EM has its values and limitations. As mentioned above, the major advantage of EM is to identify the detailed cellular organelles. Additionally, the intercellular matrix, cell–cell relationship and small areas of architectural organization may also provide diagnostic information. On the other hand, the areas examined by EM are many times smaller than those for LM. The architectural organization, so important in diagnosing sarcomas, is not as clear. Since certain diagnostic structures are not always present in all tumor cells, sampling on the so-called thick (semi-thin) sections has to be very careful. Even the cells examined by EM have to be carefully interpreted so that the non-neoplastic cells are not mistaken for representative tumor cells. Further, characteristic EM features may be absent, hence, providing no diagnostic value. Similarly, the blood vessels seen on EM may not necessarily indicate a sarcoma of vascular nature. Many non-vascular sarcomas may contain a rich vascular network. It is mandatory to evaluate the EM features along with the light microscopy and pertinent clinical data. Making an interpretation on EM alone is potentially dangerous and, therefore, an unacceptable approach.

Whether EM should be performed or not depends on how diagnostic the LM features are. For example, if a pleomorphic mesenchymal tumor shows unequivocal cross striations in some tumor cells, there is no need to confirm the diagnosis of rhabdomyosarcoma by EM. On the other hand, if the histologic and cytologic features of a spindle cell tumor are so equivocal on LM that two or more diagnoses may result, EM may then be considered.

Table 1 shows the common diagnostic problems in soft tissue sarcomas encountered by LM, which may be resolved by demonstrating characteristic EM structure(s). While most of the EM structures help establish the diagnosis or the nature of tumor cells, they may not necessarily elucidate, and in some instances, raise further questions about the histogenesis. For instance, the concept of synovial origin of clear cell sarcomas has been complicated by the findings of melanosomes and/or premelanosomes. Though the changes of nuclei and cytoplasmic organelles are more striking in malignant cells than in their normal or benign counterparts, EM features alone are usually insufficient to distinguish benign from malignant tumors.

Table 1. Common diagnostic problems for which EM may be helpful.

LM features that may be shared by different tumors	Tumors	Helpful EM features
	MFH	Histiocyte-like and fibroblast-like cells.
	Pleomorphic rhabdomyosarcoma	Banded filaments (cross striations)
	Liposarcoma	Lipoblast
1. Pleomorphic, spindle, polygonal and giant cells	Sarcoma	Intercellular junctions absent, or scanty and pooly-developed; features of individual type of sarcoma, e.g., banded filaments in rhabdomyosarcoma, etc.

Table 1. (continued)

LM features that may be shared by different tumors	Tumors	Helpful EM features
	2	
	Carcinoma	Intercellular junctions more conspicuous and well-developed; features of individual carcinoma, e.g., tono-filaments in squamous cell carcinoma, etc.
	Melanoma	Melanosomes and/or premelanosomes
	Fibrosarcoma	Abundant rough endoplasmic reticulum: convoluted nuclear membranes
1	Leiomyosarcoma	Myofilaments associated with dense bodies
	Malignant Schwannoma	Elongated cytoplasmic processes surrounded by basal lamina
2. Packed relatively uniform spindle cells	Sarcoma	Intercellular junctions few and usually poorly developed; in leiomyosarcomas, apposing dense plaques may mimick junctions; features of individual type of sarcoma
2	Carcinoma	Same as above
	Melanoma	Same as above
	Oat cell carcinoma	Neurosecretory granules: intercellular junctions
3. Small cells	Histiocytic lymphoma (reticulum cell) carcinoma)	Few cytoplasmic organelles; interdigitating plasma membranes without junctions
	Embryonal rhabdomyosarcoma	Banded filaments
	Alveolar soft part sarcoma	Rhomboid-shaped inclusions
	Melanoma	Melanosomes and/or premelanosomes
4. Alveolar pattern	Alveolar rhabdomyosarcoma	Banded filaments (cross striations)
	Paraganglioma	Neurosecretory granules

Studies on immunofluorescence of soft tissue sarcomas have been performed. One of these studies showed that only a small portion of rhabdomyosarcomas demonstrated binding to anti-skeletal muscle antibody and all the leiomyosarcomas failed to stain with anti-smooth muscle antibody [62]. Others were successful in staining the leiomyosarcoma with a different type of antibody against smooth muscle [63]. The diagnostic value of immunostaining technique remains to be determined.

Implantation of human soft tissue sarcomas into nude mice has been considered to be a possible tool to evaluate the morphology and differentiation of sarcomas [8, 64]. It has also been claimed that the collagen fibers seen in sarcomas may be useful in the classification of sarcomas [65].

Undoubtedly, EM is one of the special techniques that has been established as a diagnostic tool. Other techniques would probably add new dimensions to the understanding of soft tissue sarcomas. Whether they may be useful for diagnosis will have to await further and critical evaluation.

Grading and Staging

Grading the degree of differentiation is usually significant for those that have shown a good correlation between the degree of differentiation and clinical behavior. Sarcomas that have low cellularity, few mitoses and little pleomorphism, are regarded as low grade sarcomas. The high grade sarcomas are those that are cellular, extremely pleomorphic and show frequent mitoses. The degree of differentiation may be regarded as a parameter to correlate with prognosis in certain types of sarcomas, e.g., lipomatous sarcomas, leiomyosarcomas, etc. In others, such as rhabdomyosarcomas, grading is meaningless. The size, location, and the extent of sarcomas may all affect the outcome. Therefore, a staging system has been devised based on these factors [8, 66].

Comments

In soft tissue sarcomas, the traditional, careful observation and analysis continue to be a powerful and logical approach for developing new concepts. The most notable example is that of fibrous histiocytomas despite the fact that their histiocytic nature has not been completely confirmed. The current new tool, EM, has two major values. First, undoubtedly it helps establish a precise classification of many sarcomas which are otherwise unclassifiable on LM. Secondly, the EM structures have provided additional evidence for new thoughts in the consideration of histogenesis. The idea of implanting human sarcomas in nude mice is intriguing and may contribute to the understanding of etiology, pathogenesis, differentiation, response to treatment and behavior of sarcomas. With the rate of progress in technology, we should expect that new concepts or modification of even the well-established concepts in soft tissue sarcomas will continue to appear.

Acknowledgements

The author wishes to thank Mrs. E. Tinnell for preparing this manuscript and Dr. C.-C. Sun for her permission to use the case material for Figure 11C.

References

1. Rous P: A transmissible avian neoplasm (sarcoma of the common foul). J Exp Med 12:695–705, 1910.
2. Rous P: A sarcoma of the fowl transmissible by an agent separable from the tumor cells. J Exp Med 13:397–411, 1911.
3. Haguenau F, Beard JW: The avian sarcoma-leukosis complex; its biology and ultrastructure. In: Tumors induced by viruses: Ultrastructural studies. Volume 1 of Ultrastructure in Biological Systems, Dalton AJ, Haguenau F (eds). New York: Academic Press, 1962, pp 1–50.
4. Gyorkey F, Sinkovics JG, Gyorkey P: Electron microscopic observations on structures resembling myxovirus in human sarcomas. Cancer 27:1449–1454, 1971.
5. Eilber FR, Morton DL: Immunologic studies of human sarcomas: additional evidence suggesting an associated sarcoma virus. Cancer 26:588–596, 1970.
6. Wood WC, Morton DL: Host immune response to a common cell-surface antigen in human sarcomas. Detection by cytotoxicity tests. N Engl J Med 284:569–572, 1971.
7. Chen KTK, Hoffman KD, Hendricks EJ: Angiosarcoma following therapeutic irradiation. Cancer 44:2044–2048, 1979.
8. Hajdu SI: Pathology of Soft Tissue Tumors. Philadelphia: Lea and Febriger, 1979.
9. Hardy TJ, An T, Brown PW, Terz JJ: Postirradiation sarcoma (malignant fibrous histiocytoma) of axilla. Cancer 42:118–124, 1978.
10. Popper H, Thomas LB, Telles NC, Falk H, Selikoff IJ: Development of hepatic angiosarcoma in man induced by vinyl chloride, thorotrast and arsenic. Comparison with cases of unknown etiology. Am J Pathol 92:349–369, 1978.
11. Vianna NJ, Brady JA, Cardamone AT: Epidemiology of angiosarcoma of liver in New York State. NY State J Med 81:895–899, 1981.
12. de Silva Horta J: Effects of colloidal thorium dioxide extravasates in the subcutaneous tissues of the cervical region in man. Ann NY Acad Sci 145:776–785, 1967.
13. Ulbright TM, Santa Cruz DJ: Kaposi's sarcoma: Relationship with hematologic, lymphoid and thymic neoplasia. Cancer 47:963–973, 1981.
14. Millstein DI, Tang C-K, Campbell EW Jr: Angiosarcoma developing in a patient with neurofibromatosis (von Recklinhausen's disease). Cancer 47:950–954, 1981.
15. Stout AP, Lattes R: Tumors of the soft tissues. Atlas of Tumor Pathology, 2nd Series, Fasc 1, Washington D.C., Armed Forces Institute of Pathology, 1967.
16. Hajdu SI: The paradox of sarcomas. Acta Cytologica 24:373–383, 1980.
17. Reddick RL, Michelitch H, Triche TJ: Malignant soft tissue tumors (malignant fibrous histiocytoma, pleomorphic liposarcoma and pleomorphic rhabdomyosarcoma): An electron micro-

scopic study. Hum Pathol 10:327–343, 1979.

18. Fu Y-S, Gabbiani G, Kaye Gl, Lattes R: Malignant soft tissue tumors of probable histiocytic origin (malignant fibrous histiocytomas): General considerations and electron microscopic and tissue culture studies. Cancer 35:176–198, 1975.

19. Morales AR, Fine G, Pardo V, Horn RC Jr: The ultrastructure of smooth muscle tumors with a consideration of the possible relationship of glomangiomas, hemangiopericytomas, and cardiac myxomas. Pathol Ann 10:65–92, 1975.

20. MacKay B, Osborne BM: The contribution of electron microscopy to the diagnosis of tumors. Pathobiol Ann 8:359–405, 1978.

21. O'Brien JE, Stout AP: Malignant fibrous xanthomas. Cancer 17:1445–1455, 1964.

22. Ozzello L, Stout AP, Murray MR: Cultural characteristics of malignant histiocytomas and fibrous xanthomas. Cancer 16:331–344, 1963.

23. Kempson RL, Kyriakos M: Fibroxanthosarcoma of the soft tissues. A type of malignant fibrous histiocytoma. Cancer 29:961–976, 1972.

24. Weiss SW, Enzinger FM: Malignant fibrous histiocytoma. An analysis of 200 cases. Cancer 41:2250–2266, 1978.

25. Kearney MM, Soule EH, Ivins JC: Malignant fibrous histiocytoma. A retrospective study of 167 cases. Cancer 45:167–178, 1980.

26. Weiss SW, Enzinger FM: Myxoid variant of malignant fibrous histiocytoma. Cancer 39:1672–1685, 1977.

27. Kyriakos M, Kempson RL: Inflammatory fibrous histiocytoma. An aggressive and lethal lesion. Cancer 37:1584–1606, 1976.

28. Enzinger FM: Angiomatoid malignant fibrous histiocytoma. A distinct fibrohistiocytic tumor of children and young adults simulating a vascular neoplasm. Cancer 44:2147–2157, 1979.

29. Ozzello L, Hamels J: The histiocytic nature of dermatofibrosarcoma protuberans. Tissue culture and electron microscopic study. Am J Clin Pathol 65:136–148, 1976.

30. Churg AM, Kahn LB: Myofibroblasts and related cells in malignant fibrous and fibrohistiocytic tumors. Hum Pathol 8:205–218, 1977.

31. Enzinger FM, Harvey DA: Spindle cell lipoma. Cancer 36:1852–1859, 1975.

32. Shmookler BM, Enzinger FM: Pleomorphic lipoma: A benign tumor simulating liposarcoma. A clinicopathologic analysis of 48 cases. Cancer 47:126–133, 1981.

33. Horvat BI, Caines M, Fisher ER: The ultrastructure of rhabdomyosarcoma. Am J Clin Pathol 53:555–564, 1970.

34. Fields JP, Helwig EB: Leiomyosarcoma of the skin and subcutaneous tissue. Cancer 47:156–169, 1981.

35. Wile AG, Evans HL, Romsdahl MM: Leiomyosarcoma of soft tissue. A clinicopathologic study. Cancer 48:1022–1032, 1981.

36. Krall RA, Kostianovsky M, Patchefsky AS: Synovial sarcoma. A clinical, pathological, and ultrastructural study of 26 cases supporting the recognition of a monophasic variant. Am J Surg Pathol 5:137–151, 1981.

37. Hajdu SI, Shiu MH, Fortner JG: Tendosynovial sarcoma: A clinicopathological study of 136 cases. Cancer 39:1201–1217, 1977.

38. Alvarez-Fernandez E, Esçalona- Zapata J: Monophasic mesenchymal synovial sarcoma: Its identification by tissue culture. Cancer 47:628–635, 1981.

39. Maddox JC, Evans HL: Angiosarcoma of skin and soft tissue. A study of forty-four cases. Cancer 48:1907–1921, 1981.

40. Ongkasuwan C, Taylor JE, Tang C-K, Prempree T: Angiosarcoma of the uterus and ovary. Cancer 49:1469–1475, 1982.

41. Stewart FW, Treve N: Lymphangiosarcoma in post-mastectomy lymphedema. A report of six cases in elephantiasis chirurgica. Cancer 1:64–81, 1948.

42. Sordillo PP, Chapman R, Hajdu SI, Magill GB, Golbey RB: Lymphangiosarcoma. Cancer 48:1674–1679, 1981.
43. Rosai J, Sumner HW, Kostianovsky M, Perez-Mesa C: Angiosarcoma of the skin. A clinicopathologic and fine structural study. Hum Pathol: 7:83–109, 1976.
44. Sterry W, Steigleder G-K, Bodeux E: Kaposi's sarcoma: Venous capillary hemangioblastoma. Arch Dermatol Res 266:253–267, 1979.
45. Cox FH, Helwig EB: Kaposi's sarcoma. 12:289–298, 1959.
46. Safai B, Mike V, Giraldo G, Beth E, Good RA: Association of Kaposi's sarcoma with second primary malignancies. Possible etiopathogenic implications. Cancer 45:1472–1479, 1980.
47. Stout AP, Murray MR: Hemangiopericytoma: a vascular tumor featuring Zimmermann's pericytes. Ann Surg 116:26–33, 1942.
48. Stout AP: Hemangiopericytoma: a study of twenty-five new cases. Cancer 2:1027–1035, 1949.
49. McMaster MJ, Soule EH, Ivins JC: Hemangiopericytoma. A clinicopathologic study and long-term follow up of 60 patients. Cancer 36:2232–2244, 1975.
50. Enzinger FM, Smith BH: Hemangiopericytoma: An analysis of 106 cases. Hum Pathol 7:61–82, 1976.
51. Nunnery EW, Kahn LB, Reddick RL, Lipper S: Hemangiopericytoma: A light microscopic and ultrastructural study. Cancer 47:906–914, 1981.
52. Stout AP: Fibrosarcoma. The malignant tumor of fibroblasts. Cancer 1:30–63, 1948.
53. Taxy JB, Battifora H, Trujillo Y, Dorfman HD: Electron microscopy in the diagnosis of malignant schwannoma. Cancer 48:1381–1391, 1981.
54. Christopherson WM, Foote FW, Stewart FW: Alveolar soft part sarcoma. Structurally characteristic tumors of uncertain histogenesis. Cancer 5:100–111, 1952.
55. Fisher ER, Reidbord H: Electron microscopic evidence suggesting the myogenic derivation of the so-called soft part sarcoma. Cancer 29:150–159, 1971.
56. Unni KK, Soule EH: Alveolar soft part sarcoma. An electron microscopic study. Mayo Clin Proc 50:591–598, 1975.
57. Enzinger FM: Clear-cell sarcoma of tendons and aponeuroses. An analysis of 21 cases. Cancer 18:1163–1174, 1965.
58. Kubo T: Clear-cell sarcoma of patellar tendon studied by electron microscopy. Cancer 24:948–953, 1969.
59. Hoffman GJ, Carten D: Clear cell sarcoma of tendons and aponeuroses with melanin. Arch Pathol 95:22–25, 1973.
60. Enzinger FM: Epithelioid sarcoma: A sarcoma simulating a granuloma or a carcinoma. Cancer 26:1029–1041, 1970.
61. Patchefsky AS, Soriano R, Kostianovsky M: Epithelioid sarcoma. Ultrastructural similarity to nodular synovitis. Cancer 39:143–152, 1977.
62. Pertschuk LP: Immunofluorescence of soft-tissue tumors with anti-smooth-muscle and anti-skeletal-muscle antibodies. Am J Clin Pathol 63–332–342, 1975.
63. Bures JC, Barnes L, Mercer D: A comparative study of smooth muscle tumor utilizing light and electron microscopy, immunocytochemical staining and enzyme assay. Cancer 48:2420–2426, 1981.
64. Hajdu SI, Lemos LB, Kozakewich H, Helson L, Beattie EJ Jr: Growth pattern and differentiation of human soft tissue sarcomas in nude mice. Cancer 47:90–98, 1981.
65. Stern R: Current concepts in the diagnosis of human soft tissue sarcomas. Hum Pathol 12:777–781, 1981.
66. Russel WO, Cohen J, Enzinger FM, Hajdu SI, Heise H, Martin RG, Meissner W, Miller WT, Schmitz RL, Suit HD: A clinical and pathological staging system for soft tissue sarcomas. Cancer 40:1562–1570, 1977.

2. Diagnostic Strategy for Adult Soft Tissue Sarcomas

MICHAEL A. SIMON and LAWRENCE L. KERNS

The optimal diagnostic evaluation of the patient with a soft tissue sarcoma is designed to determine the local and distant extent of the tumor and to establish a diagnosis. If surgery alone is to be the primary mode of local treatment, the local extent of the sarcoma must be determined as accurately as possible. Notable in this regard is the importance of thorough imaging before biopsy. Not only are scintigraphy, arteriography and computed axial tomography less useful in determining local tumor extent after biopsy, but their results may well suggest other pertinent tests needed before biopsy. In this chapter we shall propose a complex diagnostic strategy for the evaluation of soft-tissue sarcomas in adults. This strategy is based on the anatomic behavior of the tumors, and includes the medical history and physical examination, scintigraphic, conventional and computed imaging, and biopsy. The rational application of these tests in an orderly fashion will yield a cost-effective and complete preoperative characterization of the sarcoma in its local and distant extent.

Anatomic Characteristics of Soft Tissue Sarcomas

Necessary to a systematic diagnostic evaluation of soft tissue sarcomas is an understanding of the local behavior and metastatic potential of this tumor class. Soft tissue sarcomas seem to arise in a single microscopic site and to grow in a centrifugal manner. Peripheral tumor cells together with bordering reactive but 'normal' tissue cells become layered and compressed, offering the gross appearance of encapsulation (Fig. 1). However, the reactive zone or host tissue, composed of inflammatory cells in a neovascularized, edematous soft tissue, is predictably but sporadically transgressed by microscopic extensions of tumor, resulting in small, extra-lesional intramuscular satellite colonies of malignant cells, well outside the boundaries of the apparent pseudocapsule (Figs. 2 and 3). Occasional rests of tumor cells may be found quite distant from the principal lesion, and probably represent extensions [1, 2, 3].

In their local growth and spread, soft tissue sarcomas are known to respect

Baker, L.H. (ed.), Soft Tissue Sarcomas. ISBN 0-89838-584-9
© *1983 Martinus Nijhoff Publishers, Boston/The Hague/Dordrecht/Lancaster. Printed in the Netherlands.*

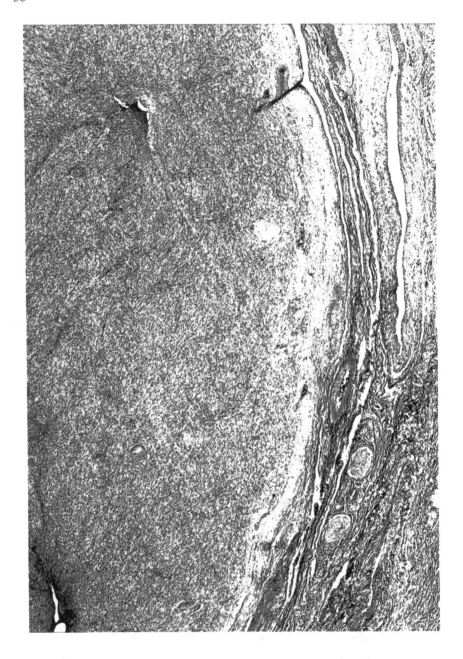

Fig. 1. A photomicrograph of a malignant fibrous histiocytoma shows the tumor on the left and its pseudocapsule on the right. Note the compressed fibrous tissue surrounding the tumor and the neovascularity adjacent to the pseudocapsule (Hematoxylin and Eosin × 20).

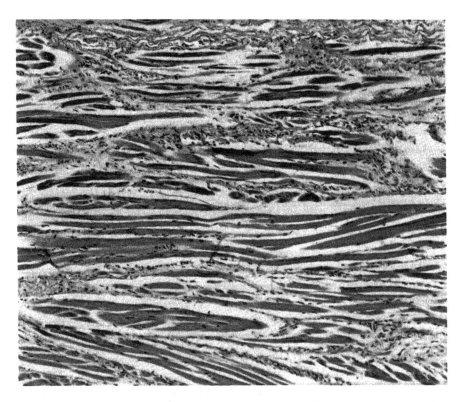

Fig. 2. A photograph of a low-grade sarcoma infiltrating muscle bundles that are longitudinally sectioned (Hematoxylin and Eosin × 100).

major fascial planes and, except late in their course or unless disrupted by surgical intervention, remain limited to a well-defined anatomic compartment (bounded by fascia, bone or articular cartilage) (Fig. 4). In contrast, tumors arising outside of a well-delimited compartment, for example, in the popliteal space or the femoral triangle, can spread greater distances without encountering anatomic barriers. Thus it is apparent that biopsy may contaminate a second anatomic compartment and facilitate tumor spread.

Major nerves and vessels are preferentially displaced rather than invaded. Metastases occur by the hematogenous route, usually to the lungs or other bones. Regional lymph node involvement, an infrequent occurrence, is prognostically equivalent to metastatic disease. Although this local anatomic and histologic conception of soft tissue sarcomas ignores the possible systemic nature of the disease, it provides a rational basis for the local treatment of these tumors as we currently understand them.

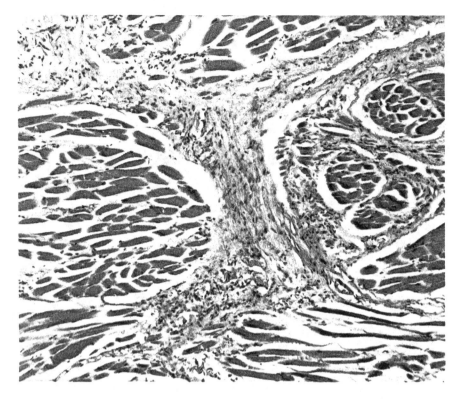

Fig. 3. A photomicrograph of a low-grade sarcoma separating muscle fascicles that are axially sectioned (Hematoxylin and Eosin × 100).

Clinical Evaluation

Evaluation begins with a careful history and physical examination. The patient usually seeks medical advice regarding a painless mass whose average duration may be over two years. No particular sex predilection has been observed, and the patient is typically twenty to sixty years of age, except for patients with synovial sarcoma who are usually twenty to forty years of age. Information should be sought regarding systemic symptoms and the patient's general state of health and suitability for operation.

Besides a thorough general physical examination, an involved extremity should be examined for muscle atrophy, decreased range of motion, and joint effusions. The mass is examined for location, size, shape, consistency, mobility, tenderness and warmth. The neurologic, arterial and venous function of the extremity should be noted, and draining lymph nodes palpated for malignant infiltration. Unless the tumor is very large and compresses venous drainage resulting in unilateral limb edema, there is no obvious vascular abnormality. It is

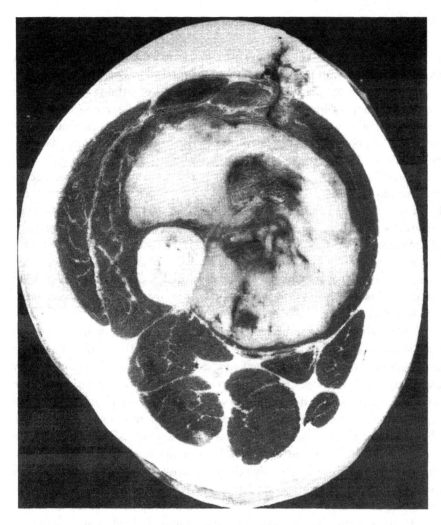

Fig. 4. A photograph of a cross section of a thigh obtained following a hip disarticulation for a soft tissue sarcoma. This photograph demonstrates that the tumor, although large, is confined to the anterior compartment of the thigh. It is contained by the medial intermuscular septum and the cortex of the femur while pushing, but not invading, the superficial femoral vessels posteriorly.

also rare to find neurologic deficits. In the case of a pelvic tumor, rectal and pelvic examinations may help in physical assessment. Baseline laboratory examination should include a complete blood count, urinalysis, erythrocyte sedimentation rate, and multiphasic serum chemistry. Occasionally the sedimentation rate and lactic dehydrogenase will be elevated with very large tumors. It must be emphasized, however, that the history and physical examination are notoriously unreliable in determining the malignancy of a soft tissue mass.

Simple Diagnostic Imaging

The radiographic evaluation begins with standard biplanar roentgenograms. Depending on the radiographic density of the mass, this can illustrate the size, anatomic site and possibly the internal characteristics of certain tumors (such as the radiolucency of lipomas or abnormal calcification of some sarcomas) [4]. Usually the mass is of water density, which is a non-diagnostic finding. Infrequently the conventional radiograph will show involvement of the bone or neighboring joint.

Xeroradiography has a wide exposure latitude, revealing simultaneous detail in bone and surrounding soft-tissues [5, 6]. The property of edge contrast enhancement helps delineate soft tissue changes and the observer can distinguish the usually smooth margins of a benign tumor from the poorly defined margins of a malignancy. Furthermore, internal structure is usually clarified and characteristics such as calcification or ossification are demonstrated. A gross estimate of size and location is possible, but false negatives are common, especially when the mass is isodense. Like the conventional radiograph, the xeroradiograph demonstrates bone involvement only late in the disease course.

Ultrasound is used in some centers as the second diagnostic modality after conventional roentgenograms for soft tissue lesions of the extremity [7]. The extremity is particularly well-suited to sonographic analysis unhampered by overlying bowel gas or thick layers of adipose tissue. Most soft tissue lesions have an acoustical impedance different from surrounding normal tissue, with distinct separating interfaces. The ability to detect these differences coupled with the ability to visualize the tissue in both transverse and longitudinal planes yields a sonogram with a clear and accurate reproduction of lesional configuration. Proponents of ultrasound argue that compared with computed tomography, it is more sensitive in detecting small tumors, more accurate in measuring tumor extent and size, and simpler to use, without radiation exposure to the patient. It is admittedly less accurate, however, in demonstrating individual muscle groups and vascular structures, especially in complex anatomic sites.

Scintigraphic Imaging

Technetium-99m phosphonate bone scanning has a limited role in the preoperative staging of soft-tissue sarcomas. Highly vascular tumors may themselves show increased soft tissue scintigraphic intensity, especially in the early 'blood pool' images, and distant metastases to bone will usually be apparent.

An additional value of the image is in local staging, where increased focal intensity in neighboring bone suggests actual bone invasion [8, 9]. In cases where the bone is radiographically normal, but diffusely hot on scan, the pathological specimen will infrequently demonstrate tumor invasion of bone, but the reactive tissue zone between lesion and bone is very narrow. Enneking found bone scans to be 92% accurate in determining bone involvement by soft tissue sarcoma, where bone involvement was defined as the contiguous relationship of bone to the tumor or its surrounding reactive tissue as verified by the pathologic specimen [8].

Gallium-67 citrate scan can be diagnostically useful in identifying occult non-pulmonary metastases and in distinguishing sarcomas from benign, non-inflammatory conditions [9]. Almost all soft tissue sarcomas as well as inflammatory masses will show increased scintigraphic activity whereas most benign non-inflammatory masses show no increase in tracer activity. Neither gallium scanning nor bone scanning has proven useful in determining the local extra-osseous extent of tumor.

Complex Diagnostic Imaging

Computed axial tomography is particularly helpful in delimiting the local extent of soft tissue tumors [10, 11]. Computed tomography detects tissue density differences between the tumor and the surrounding normal muscle, fascia or bone. Also detected are gross distortions of the normal anatomy. Visualization of neighboring vessels is enhanced by intravenous or intra-arterial injection of contrast material during the scan. Surgical and pathologic correlation with preoperative computed tomography have proven it extremely accurate in delineating the cross-sectional or transverse extent of tumor, including its relation to muscle, soft tissue and bone [12]. Unfortunately the longitudinal extent is not as reliably predicted, due to the necessity of estimating the proximal and distal borders within the 'thickness' of the terminal 'cuts.' Identification of soft tissue masses and characterization of borders as infiltrative or pseudocapsular is usually possible with computed tomography, but false negatives have been obtained, especially when the tumor is small, isodense, or non-disruptive to the normal anatomy [7]. This modality is perhaps most useful in areas of complex anatomy, such as the pelvis, retroperitoneum, shoulder girdle, or proximal thigh. However, isodense masses are fairly common, making difficult the discrimination of tumor from muscle.

Selective biplanar angiography also has a prominent role in the preoperative staging of soft tissue tumors. Although it cannot reliably distinguish benign from malignant masses, it effectively delineates the extraosseous extent of tumor and, better than any other available technique, outlines the vascular anatomy of the tumor and identifies encasement or invasion of major vessels [13, 14]. Biplanar views obtained by an experienced radiologist well apprised of the clinical information will demonstrate the relationship of tumor to major arteries in the early arterial phase. Views during midphase should show the blush of the tumor mass and possibly arteriovenous shunting. The late venous phase localizes the principal draining veins, whose intraoperative control can minimize tumor embolization. Results of arteriography in the pelvis, trunk and shoulder girdle may be disappointing, and computed tomography is more useful in these areas.

Detection of Regional or Distant Disease

The regional extent of disease is occasionally clarified by lymphangiogram, intravenous pyelogram or barium study of the colon. Other than childhood rhabdomyosarcoma and synovial sarcoma, soft tissue sarcomas rarely spread to lymph nodes, and such spread if present is equivalent to metastatic disease. Lymphangiography will occasionally demonstrate regional lymph node metastases but false positives are commonplace, especially in the inguinal and femoral node groups. Physical examination is probably more specific than any diagnostic imaging for the detection of regional lymph node metastases.

Primary sarcomas in the pelvis or retroperitoneum may well exert local compressive or displacement effects on the genitourinary or lower gastrointestinal tracts. In these cases, the intravenous pyelogram and barium enema may be helpful in delineating the anatomy and possible impingement of the tumor.

Assessment of the extent of disseminated disease completes the prebiopsy staging evaluation. Distant spread of soft tissue sarcoma most frequently involves lung, and secondly bone. The technetium-99m phosphonate bone scan as described above is a sufficient screen for bone metastases. The detection of pulmonary metastases is possible by conventional roentgenogram, conventional tomography and computed axial tomography in order of increasing sensitivity. The conventional chest roentgenogram will visualize relatively large lesions only, and conventional tomography is more sensitive and usually more helpful. Computed axial tomography is more sensive even than conventional tomography and is especially successful in demonstrating pleural based lesions [15]. Its great sensitivity however results in many false positives, i.e., lesions found at thoracotomy to be inflammatory rather than malignant. At this time it is difficult to compare the results of a plethora of computed scanning instruments, but it is likely that computed axial tomography will play the dominant role in pulmonary imaging in the future.

Biopsy

Biopsy is the last but most important step in diagnosis before operation [16]. The clinical, radiographic and scintigraphic evaluation of soft tissue sarcomas, though critical to the determination of local and distant tumor extent, are only preliminary to biopsy, the key diagnostic study. A tissue diagnosis must be obtained by biopsy prior to definitive treatment. Furthermore, the biopsy should be performed by the surgeon who will ultimately provide the definitive surgical treatment, and should be neither left to inexperienced assistants nor obtained by the primary practitioner before referral. Performance of the biopsy should be the culmination of a carefully orchestrated battery of diagnostic tests whose results help determine the appropriate site for biopsy, the need for open rather than closed biopsy or excisional rather than incisional biopsy, the advisability of using a tourniquet, the usefulness of frozen section analysis or special tissue studies, and the possibility for immediate operative treatment.

We recommend complete clinical, roentgenographic, and scintigraphic staging before biopsy for three reasons: 1) data obtained may change the differential diagnosis before biopsy allowing a more accurate clinicopathologic correlation and providing a more solid foundation for definitive diagnosis at biopsy, 2) the aforementioned staging tests are less useful for determining local extent of disease after disruption of tissue planes, hematoma formation and wound healing, and 3) complete pre-biopsy staging allows frozen section analysis of the tissue specimen followed immediately by definitive operative treatment if so desired. Furthermore, if the surgeon is prepared to do immediate surgery, he is more likely to place the biopsy incision appropriately.

The key element in the biopsy of a soft tissue mass is the correct placement of the biopsy incision. Choice of the biopsy site should be based on the pre-biopsy differential diagnosis and the extent of the primary tumor as predicted by clinical staging. With this information and understanding of the principles of limb-salvage procedures and standard and non-standard amputation flaps, the surgeon can formulate an operative plan and place the biopsy incision in a site amenable to *en-bloc* resection with any of the likely definitive operations.

The surgeon must weigh the relative advantages and disadvantages of open versus closed biopsy. Closed biopsy by needle leaves a small puncture wound which is easily excised at operation. There is also usually less hematoma, less likelihood of infection and greater ease of performance in the minor surgery suite. The greatest disadvantage of closed biopsy is the relatively 'blind' acquisition of a small amount of tissue which results in a significant incidence of inadequate tissue sample and a decreased overall accuracy. Open biopsy, on the other hand, requires an incision sufficient for exposure and dissection within the tumor-affected compartment, carrying the increased risks, complications and consequences of incorrect placement. The hematoma can be sizeable and tumor spillage significant. However, the tissue sample obtained is as large as necessary for pathologic diagnosis and a representative area can be selected under direct vision. Open biopsy remains the preferred technique in most centers.

Helpful guidelines for the incision placement in the extremities include use of a

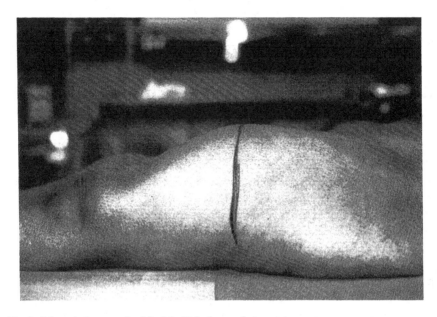

Fig. 5. A lateral photograph of the left thigh shows a large mass.

longitudinal rather than a transverse incision which is more difficult to excise, avoidance of major neurovascular structures lest they be damaged or needlessly contaminated, and caution against penetration of deep major compartments other than those involved with tumor. A scalpel should be used throughout the procedure, with care taken not to crush the specimen. The smallest incision compatible with an adequate tissue sample is appropriate. The most viable, representative and diagnostic tissue is found at the margin of the tumor-pseudo-capsule interface. As the lesion is approached the muscle color will change from red to salmon, and the tumor itself will appear gray or white. It is best to avoid any irradiated tissue and the necrotic tumor center as they will prove non-diagnostic. Lastly, of utmost importance are careful hemostasis and meticulous closure. For extremity lesions, a tourniquet affords better visualization of the field and facilitates a rapid and bloodless procedure. However, the limb should not be exsanguinated by compression, risking tumor cell embolization, and the tourniquet should be released and hemostasis obtained prior to skin closure.

Soft tissue specimens should be submitted for frozen section analysis regardless of whether or not immediate surgery is planned. This ensures an adequate and representative sample for pathologic analysis. The advantages of immediate surgery can be gained if the diagnosis of the frozen section is consistent with the prebiopsy staging evaluation. Thus the patient can be spared one anesthetic exposure, the biopsy hematoma is reduced, and the theoretical possibility of diminishing the systemic spread of a malignant neoplasm remains.

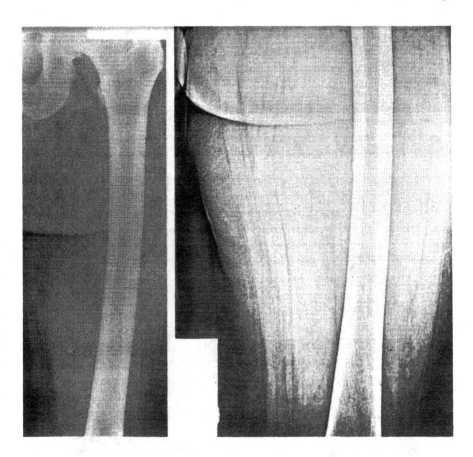

Fig. 6. (left). Conventional roentgenogram of the left thigh shows a water-density mass that is ill-defined, without internal calcification. No femoral involvement is visible.

Fig. 7 (right). Xeroradiogram of the left thigh shows a water density mass that is somewhat better defined than in the conventional roentgenogram. It also shows that the mass is homogeneous, without internal calcification, and does not involve the femur.

Case Example

The following case example illustrates the optimal diagnostic strategy for a soft tissue sarcoma (Figs. 5–14). A healthy sixty-year-old black woman complained of a painless, rapidly growing mass in the left thigh for three months. Physical examination showed a large, moderately mobile mass that was located beneath the deep fascia in the left anterior thigh (Fig. 5). The neurovascular and regional lymph node examination were normal. A conventional roentgenogram revealed a water-density mass without any calcification (Fig. 6). The xerogram showed a homogeneous, partially well-defined mass that was of water density without

40

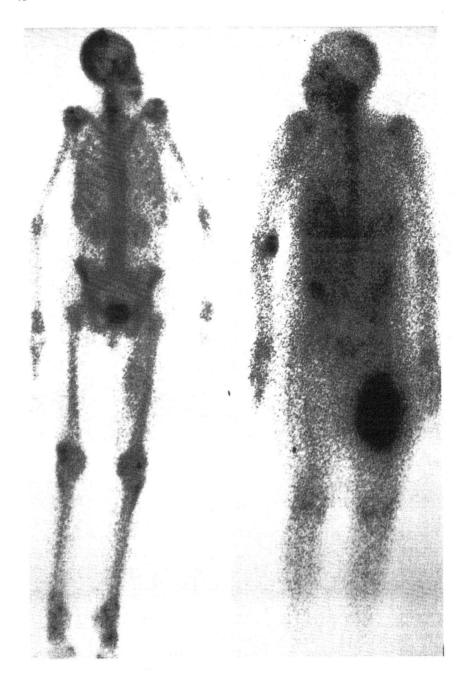

Fig. 8 (left). Technetium-99m phosphonate total-body scan demonstrates soft-tissue uptake of the tracer, but osseous structures are normal except for some probable osteoarthritis of the great toes.

Fig. 9 (right). Gallium-67 citrate scan demonstrates an intense scintigraphic activity only at the site of the primary tumor. The tracer activity at the right elbow is at the site of injection of the tracer.

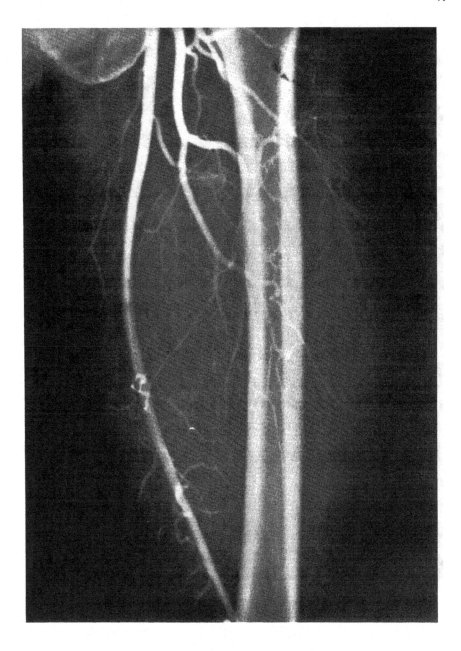

Fig. 10. Early phase of the peripheral angiogram demonstrates medial displacement of the superficial femoral artery.

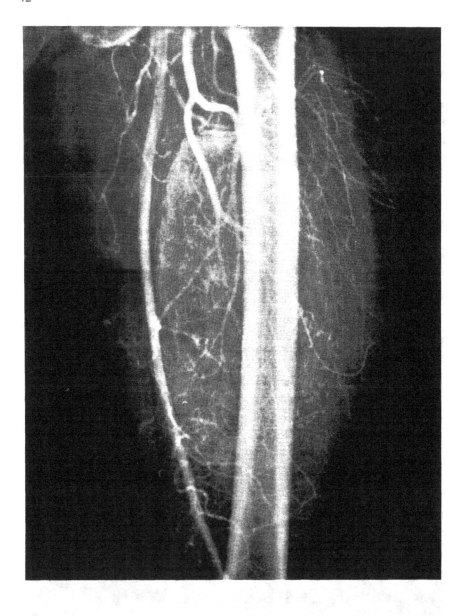

Fig. 11. Mid-phase of the peripheral angiogram also demonstrates the displacement of the superficial femoral artery and shows that the tumor is very vascular, being supplied primarily by branches
from the deep femoral artery. There are numerous 'tumor' vessels.

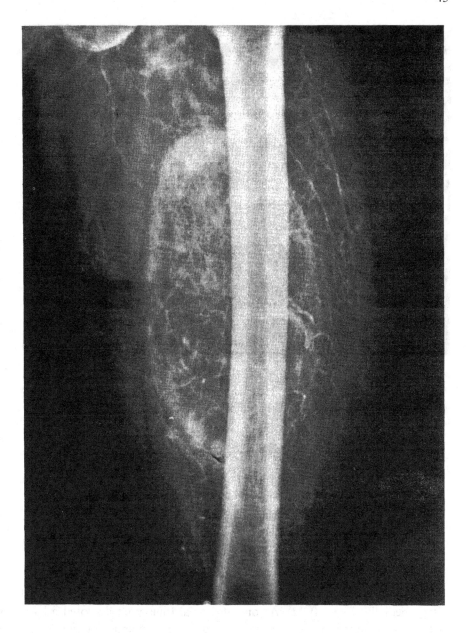

Fig. 12. Venous phase of the arteriogram demonstrates an extensive venous flush even when the major veins can no longer be visualized. There is obvious venous pooling.

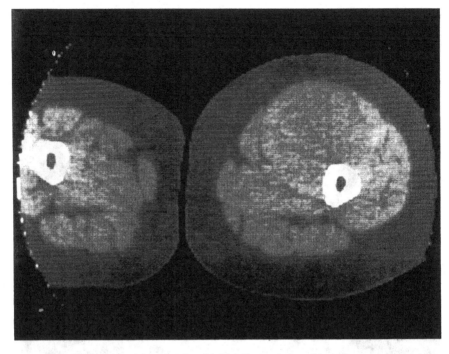

Fig. 13. Computed axial tomogram of the mid-thigh shows a lesion with almost the same density as the muscle in the anterior-medial aspect of the thigh, in the quadriceps muscle overlying the diaphysis of the femur, and displacing the superficial femoral artery medially.

calcification (Fig. 7). The clinician was confident that this was a malignant soft tissue mass and instituted diagnostic and staging evaluation for a malignant soft-tissue tumor.

A technetium-99m phosphonate bone scan showed only soft tissue uptake in the area of the known tumor (Fig. 8); there were no bone lesions. A gallium-67 citrate scan showed very intense scintigraphic activity at the site of the mass, but no other abnormalities, a finding consistent with a primary soft-tissue sarcoma (Fig. 9).

In the angiogram, a highly vascular mass displaced the superficial femoral artery medially (Figs. 10–12). A computed axial tomogram disclosed a large water-density mass in the substance of the quadriceps muscle anterior to and lying against the diaphysis of the femur, displacing the superficial femoral artery posterior-medially (Fig. 13). The conventional chest roentgenogram and computed tomogram of the lungs showed no evidence of metastases.

The diagnostic and imaging tests confirmed the clinician's impression that the tumor was malignant. The surgeon performed an incisional biopsy. On frozen section analysis a high-grade sarcoma was found. The surgeon had decided

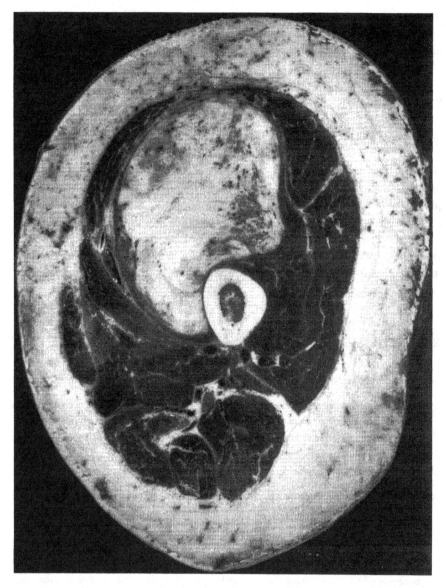

Fig. 14. An axial section of the surgical specimen at the mid-thigh shows the tumor to be in the substance of the vastus medialis, lying against the surface of the femur and displacing the superficial vessels medially.

beforehand to perform a surgical procedure that had radical margins under these circumstances. The only operation which could predictively achieve this goal was a hip disarticulation. This was done during the same anesthesia.

An axial section of the surgical specimen confirmed the findings of the imaging studies (Fig. 14). The tumor was in the substance of the vastus medialis, lying on the periosteum of the femur and displacing the superficial femoral vessels medially and posteriorly. The final microscopic diagnosis was a malignant fibrous histiocytoma.

Summary

In summary, the diagnostic evaluation of the patient with a soft tissue sarcoma entails a complex strategy designed to demonstrate the local and distant extent of tumor prior to obtaining tissue diagnosis. Evaluation begins with the medical history, physical examination, and conventional roentgenogram. Next employed is a carefully planned sequence of diagnostic imaging methods as discussed above. Lastly undertaken is the technically simple, but conceptually complex biopsy. As cannot be overemphasized, a single responsible and experienced surgeon is crucial to direct and analyze the pre-biopsy staging evaluation, to plan and execute a biopsy designed to diagnose the disease without compromising the cure, and to complete the definitive surgical treatment.

References

1. Simon MA, Spanier SS, Enneking WF: Management of adult soft-tissue sarcomas of the extremities. Surg Annu 11:363–402, 1979.
2. Simon MA, Enneking WF: The management of soft-tissue sarcomas of the extremities. J Bone Joint Surg 58-A:317–327, 1976.
3. Enneking WF, Spanier SS, Malawer MM: The effect of the anatomic setting on the results of surgical procedures for soft parts sarcoma of the thigh. Cancer 47:1005–1022, 1981.
4. Martel W, Abell MR: Radiographic evaluation of soft tissue tumors. Cancer 32:352–366, 1973.
5. Wolfe JN: Xeroradiography of bones, joints and soft tissues. Radiology 93:583–587, 1969.
6. Wolfe JN: Xeroradiography: image content and comparison with film roentgenograms. Am J Roentgenol Radium Ther Nucl Med 117:690–695, 1973.
7. Bernardino ME, Jing B, Thomas JL, Lindell MM, Zornoza J: The extremity soft-tissue lesion: a comparative study of ultrasound, computed tomography and xeroradiography. Radiology 139:53–59, 1981.
8. Enneking WF, Chew FS, Springfield DS, Hudson TM, Spanier SS: The role of radionuclide bone-scanning in determining the resectability of soft-tissue sarcomas. J Bone Joint Surg 63/A:249–257, 1981.
9. Kirchner PT, Simon MA: Clinical utility of bone and gallium scanning of soft tissue masses (in press).
10. Berger PE, Kuhn JP: Computed tomography of tumors of the musculoskeletal system in children. Radiology 127:171–175, 1978.
11. De Santos LA, Goldstein HM, Murray JA, Wallace S: Computed tomography in the evaluation of musculoskeletal neoplasm. Radiology 128:89–94, 1978.
12. Heelan RT, Watson RC, Smith J: Computed tomography of lower extremity tumors. AJR 132:933–937, 1979.
13. Hudson TM, Haas G, Enneking WF, Hawkins IF: Angiography in the management of mus-

culoskeletal tumors. Surg. Gynecol Obstet 141:11–21, 1975.

14. Levin DC, Watson RC, Baltaxe HA: Arteriography in diagnosis and management of acquired peripheral soft-tissue masses. Radiology 103:53–58, 1972.

15. Chang AE, Schaner EG, Conkle DM, Flye MW, Doppman JL, Rosenberg SA: Evaluation of computed tomography in the detection of pulmonary metastases: a prospective study. Cancer 43:913–916, 1979.

16. Simon MA: Biopsy of Musculoskeletal tumors. J Bone Joint Surg 64A:1253–1257, 1982.

3. Staging of Soft Tissue Sarcomas

JAMES R. RYAN

It is important to stage malignant neoplasms in order to be able to: (1) plan a rational program of therapy, (2) compare comparable lesions and various methods of treatment in end result studies. The first staging system for malignant neoplasms was designed for carcinoma of the cervix. This was first undertaken by the League of Nations and then revised in the 'Annual Report on the Results of Treatment in Carcinoma of the Uterus'. Since then, many staging systems for different neoplasms have been designed. Because of their small numbers and numerous histological types, a clinical staging system for sarcomas was not attempted until recently. It has been suggested that histologic type is not as important as histologic grading in soft tissue sarcomas and, consequently, all soft tissue sarcomas could be grouped together to allow sufficient numbers to formulate a staging system. A Task Force was appointed in 1968 by The American Joint Committee for Cancer Staging and End Results Reporting to devise a staging system for sarcomas of soft tissue. They utilized the TNM system devised by the Union Internationale Contre le Cancere – T standing for tumor and recorded by size or with local invasion of nerves, blood vessels or bone; N for lymph node involvement; and M for metastases. They also felt that grade was important and added this component to their staging system, thus, evaluating four characteristics of soft tissue sarcomas (Table 1). This staging system has not been found useful by most surgical oncologists. It is rather cumbersome with four items to evaluate and nine different stages. Tumor size per se should not dictate surgical treatment. Regional lymph node involvement in most series of soft tissue sarcomas has resulted in a poor prognosis and should probably be evaluated the same as distant metastases. Stage IV, by their criteria, may not have regional lymph node involvement but invades bone or neurovascular structures and is, therefore, relegated to a poorer prognostic sign than their Stage IIIc which has regional lymph node involvement. Involvement of bone and/or neurovascular structures may require a different surgical procedure but does not carry the same poor prognosis as does nodal involvement. Finally, their histological grading system allows for three grades – a low, moderate, and high grade microscopic appearance. Once a soft tissue sarcoma is labeled a Grade 2,

Baker, L.H. (ed.), Soft Tissue Sarcomas. ISBN 0-89838-584-9

the pressure is removed from the pathologist and the burden is placed entirely upon the surgeon as to what surgical procedure to employ.

Hajdu has developed a staging system for soft tissue sarcomas which is useful as a medical staging system and as a prognostic indicator. He utilizes tumor size, site, and histologic grade (Table 2). His grading system differentiates only

Table 1. Schema for staging soft tissue sarcomas by T, N, M and G.

T	Primary tumor	
	T_1 Tumor less than 5 cm	
	T_2 Tumor 5 cm or greater	
	T_3 Tumor that grossly invades bone, major vessel, or major nerve	
N	Regional lymph nodes	
	N_0 No histologically verified metastases to regional lymph nodes	
	N_1 Histologically verified regional lymph node metastasis	
M	Distant metastasis	
	M_0 No distant metastasis	
	M_1 Distant metastasis	
G	Histologic grade of malignancy	
	G_1 Low	
	G_2 Moderate	
	G_3 High	
Stage I		
Ia	$G_1T_1N_0M_0$	Grade 1 tumor less than 5 cm in diameter with no regional lymph nodes or distant metastases
Ib	$G_1T_2N_0M_0$	Grade 1 tumor 5 cm or greater in diameter with no regional lymph nodes or distant metastases
Stage II		
IIa	$G_2T_1N_0M_0$	Grade 2 tumor less than 5 cm in diameter with no regional lymph nodes or distant metastases
IIb	$G_2T_2N_0M_0$	Grade 2 tumor 5 cm or greater in diameter with no regional lymph nodes or distant metastases
Stage III		
IIIA	$G_3T_1N_0M_0$	Grade 3 tumor less than 5 cm in diameter with no regional lymph nodes or distant metastases
IIIc	Any $GT_{1-2}N_1M_0$	Tumor of any grade or size (no invasion) with regional lymph nodes but no distant metastases
Stage IV		
IVa	Any $GT_3N_{0-1}M_0$	Tumor of any grade that grossly invades bone, major vessel, or major nerve with or without regional lymph node metastases but without distant metastases
IVb	Any $GTNM_1$	Tumor with distant metastases

between low and high grades. He defines site as superficial or deep. This system has limited usefulness for surgical staging as tumor size and site (superficial or deep) are not reliable criteria to determine what surgical procedure to employ.

Enneking has devised a surgical staging system of musculoskeletal sarcomas which is designed for both bony and soft tissue sarcomas. His system has proven to be very useful in that it is simple while at the same time evaluates those elements that are important in the ability to plan the correct surgical procedure for soft tissue sarcomas. His system utilizes histologic grade, anatomical location and distant metastases. Three stages are then assigned – Stage I being low grade, Stage II being high grade, and Stage III being any grade with metastases. Stages I and II are subdivided into A and B by anatomical location. Stages I-A and II-A are anatomically within one compartment. Stages I-B and II-B are extracompartmental, i.e., in more than one anatomical compartment. The grading system allows for only a low grade or high grade histologic type (Table 3). By utilizing this staging system after appropriate preoperative workup, the proper surgical procedure may be selected.

Table 2. Hajdu's staging system

	Good prognostic signs	Bad prognostic signs
Size	Small	Big
	– less than 5 cm	– more than 5 cm
Site	Superficial	Deep
	– not beyond superficial fascia	– beyond superficial fascia
Histologic grade	Low	High
	– hypocellular	– hypercellular
	– much stroma	– minimal stroma
	– minimal necrosis	– much necrosis
	– good maturation	– poor maturation
	– mitosis $<5/10$ HPF	– mitosis $>5/10$ HPF

Table 3. Enneking's surgical staging system.

Stage I-A	Low grade intracompartmental lesion without metastases
Stage I-B	Low grade extracompartmental lesion without metastases
Stage II-A	High grade intracompartmental lesion without metastases
Stage II-B	High grade extracompartmental lesion without metastases
Stage III	Any grade with metastasis

52

References

1. American Joint Committee for Cancer Staging and End Results Reporting: Manual for Staging of Cancer, Chicago, American Joint Committee, 1977, pp 1-3.
2. Annual Report on the Results of Treatment in Carcinoma of the Uterus. H.L. Kottmeier, ed., Vol. 2, Stockholm, Norstedt and Söner, 1958.
3. Enneking WF, Spanier SS, Goodman MA: Current concepts review. The surgical staging of musculoskeletal sarcoma. J Bone Joint Surg 62-A:1027-1030, 1980.
4. Hajdu SI: Pathology of Soft Tissue Tumors. Philadelphia: Lea and Febiger, 1979.
5. Russell WO, Cohen J, Enzinger F, Hajdu SI, Heise H, Martin RG, Meissner W, Miller WT, Schmitz RL, Suit HD: A clinical and pathological staging system for soft tissue sarcomas. Cancer 40:1562-1570, 1977.

4. Surgical Treatment of Soft Tissue Sarcomas

JAMES R. RYAN

Numerous combined modality treatments for adult soft tissue sarcomas are presently being undertaken. It is the assumption that this will allow for local resection of soft tissue sarcomas with the same or less local recurrence rate than radical resection. Some of the multiple modality treatment programs include intra-arterial preoperative limb perfusion using most commonly adriamycin or cis-platinum, preoperative or postoperative radiotherapy, preoperative and/or postoperative chemotherapy, and tubes inserted into the wound post local resection for radium implantation. These techniques are as yet experimental and unproven and this chapter deals with the premise that complete surgical ablation of the sarcoma is the planned procedure.

Simon, *et al.* have described five surgical procedures that are available in the treatment of any sarcoma: (1) incisional biopsy, gross tumor is left; (2) excisional biopsy, microscopic tumor may be left; (3) wide local resection, microscopic tumor or skip metastases may be left; (4) radical resection (complete compartmental resection); and (5) amputation (Table 1). It is important to define the exact surgical procedure for end result studies as what was frequently described as a radical resection by the surgeon was, in fact, a wide local resection. Surgeons have probably done themselves a disservice by using the term 'radical resection'. The definition meant by surgeons is 'designed to remove the root of the disease or all diseased tissue'. Another definition of radical is extreme or drastic which is the definition assumed by most non-surgeons. Consequently, to most non-surgeons, an amputation is a radical procedure, however, it may encompass any of the other four surgical procedures depending upon the location of the amputation (i.e., an amputation through the tumor would be an incisional biopsy).

The surgeon's aim in the treatment of soft tissue sarcoma is complete eradication of the sarcoma while at the same time preserving maximum function of the extremity. The surgeon may technically be able to completely remove a soft tissue sarcoma of the foot with a radical resection, however, the patient may better be served with a below-knee amputation for function. While staging and type of surgical procedure have become standardized, evaluation of postoperative function has not. Postoperative function is frequently the biased opinion

Baker, L.H. (ed.), Soft Tissue Sarcomas. ISBN 0-89838-584-9

Table 1. Surgical procedures (Simon, et al.).

Incisional biopsy	Incisional biopsy	– Diagnosis
Excisional biopsy	Excisional biopsy	– Palliative
Wide local resection	Wide local resection	– Stage Ia
Radical resection	Radical resection	– Stage IIa
(Compartmental amputation)	Amputation	– Stage Ib
Amputation		Stage IIb

of the surgeon. We are, consequently, in the process of developing a postoperative psychological and functional index for evaluation of end results.

Once the preoperative workup has been obtained, the sarcoma may be staged and the proper surgical procedure then selected. In general, an incisional biopsy is utilized for the definitive diagnosis. An excisional biopsy may be selected for palliative treatment. Wide local resection may be indicated in Stage Ia lesions, and radical resection in Stage IIa lesions. Stage Ib and IIb sarcomas usually require amputation (Table 2). The surgeon must plan for complete eradication of the sarcoma at the time of the definitive surgical procedure. Local recurrence leads to dire consequences more than doubling the incidence of metastatic disease.

The definitive surgical procedure should be planned if possible at the time of biopsy; the biopsy wound being carefully closed and sealed and the extremity then being redraped utilizing new gowns and gloves and new instruments so as not to contaminate the operative field with tumor cells. If a diagnosis cannot be made at the time of frozen section then the wound should be closed utilizing meticulous hemostasis so as not to spread tumor cells through wound hematoma which might prevent the ability to do a radical resection or require a more proximal amputation. If the sarcoma is near a joint, the joint should be opened and inspected to ensure that tumor has not extended into the joint. If tumor has extended into the joint, the wound should be closed, these instruments discarded with plans to completely excise the joint en bloc with the rest of the resection or amputate. Each case must be considered separately and the surgical procedure planned dependent upon the patient's age, functional abilities, and location of the tumor. If resection is the planned surgical procedure for a Stage Ia lesion, a wide local resection may be considered. An arbitrary figure of three centimeters of normal margins is recommended. In Stage I fibrosarcomas and liposarcomas lesser margins may be desired as these sarcomas tend to be locally recurrent rather than metastatic in nature. Since soft tissue sarcomas tend to spread proximally and distally through fascial planes, Stage IIa lesions will require a compartmental resection or amputation. From the preoperative staging, one must decide if and what muscles, nerves, blood vessels or bones require excision and if their excision will allow for adequate function with or without reconstructive procedures. For muscle resection it must be decided if the patient can function adequately without that muscle group or if tendon transfers can be utilized to substitute for the removed muscle or if arthrodesis or bracing will allow for adequate function. If nerve must be resected the extent of resection is usually so great that repair of the nerve cannot be undertaken. It must be decided that sensory loss will not be too great to allow for function of the extremity. One must also determine that the muscle loss secondary to denervation will be acceptable or correctable by tendon transfer, arthrodesis, or bracing. If the major blood vessels to the extremity must be sacrificed, one must plan an adequate soft tissue bed for vascular grafting. Bone resection may be handled by several alternatives. In the lower leg or forearm the extremity may be converted to a phocomelia. Bone replacement may be undertaken by autograft or allograft. Autologous bone grafting has the advantage of utilizing the patient's own tissues. The major disadvantages are the amount of bone available for grafting and if joint resection is required, arthrodesis is usually necessary. Allografts have the advantage of replacing entire joints. The disadvantages of allografting are delayed healing, a possible immunological response (however, true rejection is not definable at the present time), and the possibility of virus infection. Also, an allograft bank is quite expensive. If joints must be sacrificed, the surgeon must decide upon leaving the joint flail, arthrodesing the joint, or performing an arthroplasty either utilizing bone allograft or a joint replacement. Implants for joint replacement in sarcoma surgery have generally been modifications of standard total joint replacement arthroplasties. The amount of bone necessarily removed in sarcoma surgery and the young age of the patient may make for difficult fixation and eventual loosening of the component which must be considered when utilizing this technique. Also, the muscles which must be included in the resection must be considered if there is to be a functional, movable joint postoperatively. The surgeon must weigh the results of a complete resection of a compartment in relation to the structures present in that compartment as to final functional results. If one has planned an amputation as the operative procedure of choice, it would be necessary for lesions of the foot or hand to amputate below the knee or below the elbow; for lesions of the lower leg or forearm, to amputate above the knee or above the elbow; for lesions of the distal thigh or distal arm to disarticulate at the hip or shoulder and for lesions of the proximal thigh or shoulder region, to undertake a hemipelvectomy or forequarter amputation. Numerous surgical textbooks contain descriptions of amputative techniques. In sarcoma amputation surgery, modifications are frequently needed depending upon the specific location of the sarcoma with flaps devised to avoid tissue overlying the sarcoma.

RADICAL RESECTION IN SPECIFIC ANATOMICAL LOCATIONS

Lower Extremity

Foot and Ankle

Most sarcomas of the foot or ankle would be better served functionally with a Syme, or below-knee amputation, than a radical resection.

Lower Leg

Anterior Compartment. The anterior and peroneal compartments along with the superficial and deep peroneal nerve and anterior tibial vessels may be resected with frequently good functional results. There is loss of sensation on the dorsum of the foot, however, plantar sensation is intact. The muscle loss may be handled by transfer of the posterior tibial tendon to the dorsum of the foot or by bracing, either a double upright short-leg brace with a ninety degree downstop or a plastic orthosis. If the fibula shows evidence of involvement, it may be resected with little functional loss. If the tibia is involved, bone grafting is necessary. If the

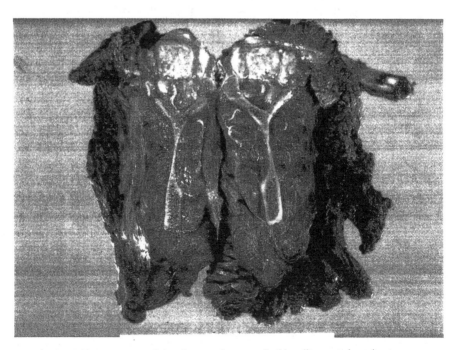

Fig. 1A. Stage IIa sarcoma overlying the scapula as seen in this split-resected specimen.

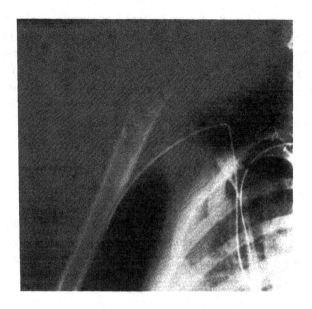

Fig. 1B. Radiograph of postoperative modified Tikhoff–Linberg resection.

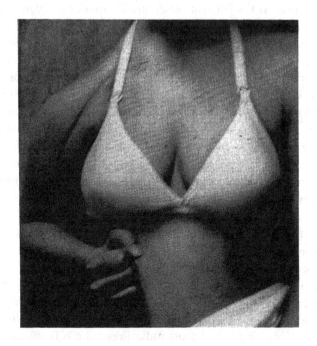

Fig. 1C. Postoperative appearance with full hand and elbow function.

fibula has remained intact, it may be fused proximally and distally to the remaining tibia with a fibular bone graft from the other leg used to replace the diaphyseal tibial resection. If both the tibia and fibula must be removed, just a fibular bone graft from the opposite extremity probably will not afford sufficient strength to prevent fracture. Allograft cadaver bone has been recommended by some surgeons to replace large cortical defects. One must weigh the anticipated long-term results of expected bony union and eventual strength when undertaking any of these procedures with the expected results of an above-knee amputation with prosthetic fitting.

Posterior Compartment. Resection of the posterior compartment of the lower leg with resection of the posterior tibial nerve and vessels results in great functional loss. There is complete loss of sensation on the plantar aspect of the foot which usually results in trophic ulcers and secondary infections. Above-knee amputation generally would provide better functional results than radical resection in this location.

Thigh

Anterior Compartment. The anterior compartment may be resected along with the femoral nerve. If the femoral vessels are involved, one might consider vascular grafting after resection. The hamstring tendons may be transferred anteriorly to assist in knee extension and the patient may be braced for lack of extension power. An arthrodesis of the knee may be undertaken, however, most people prefer to have knee joint motion preserved. If a portion of cortical bone or a diaphyseal segment of the femur must be resected because of involvement, bone reconstruction must again be undertaken utilizing either autogenous or allogenic grafts, again, recognizing the problems with bony union and strength postoperatively. If the knee joint is involved, it must be resected. Arthrodesis may then be undertaken utilizing either a turn-down bone graft from the femur or a turn-up bone graft from the tibia to achieve arthrodesis. Arthroplasty, utilizing a total knee joint may be considered, however, again, one must be concerned with possible loosening in a young patient. Allograft replacement with preservation of knee function is another consideration. If the hip joint is involved, it must be resected. The surgeon must then decide whether to leave the hip as a hanging hip type of procedure, arthrodesis with shortening of the extremity, allograft replacement, or prosthetic replacement of the hip joint with a total hip procedure. One must consider the risks of possible infection in such a large operative procedure and eventual prosthetic loosening when undertaking prosthetic arthroplasty. Obtaining an adequate radical resection is frequently difficult in sarcomas of the proximal anterior thigh. If the tumor has extended through the femoral canal into the pelvis, obviously a radical resection would not be adequate.

Posterior Compartment. Radical resection of the posterior compartment will result in resection of the sciatic nerve with complete loss of muscle power below the knee and, again, loss of sensation on the plantar aspect of the foot. Such great functional loss would result that hip disarticulation or hemipelvectomy would probably be a preferred surgical procedure.

Buttock

Sarcomas in the buttock region are difficult and generally require a hemipelvectomy. Bowden described a method of resection for sarcomas of the buttocks which he termed 'buttectomy', however, on review of these cases including thirty-six operative procedures, there was a thirty-nine percent local recurrence rate in contrast to their hemipelvectomies in which there was an eighteen percent recurrence rate. Hemipelvectomy is, therefore, generally necessary for buttock lesions.

Upper Extremity

Hand

Soft tissue sarcomas are uncommon in the hand. If one finger is involved a Ray resection may be undertaken. If the thenar eminence is the primary site, radical resection with later reconstruction is preferable to any prosthetic device. It is tempting to the surgeon to salvage as much of the hand as possible, however, he must not do this at the expense of complete surgical removal of the sarcoma.

Forearm

Posterior Compartment. The posterior compartment may be excised along with the radial nerve. Sensation will be lost on the dorsal lateral aspect of the hand. Tendon transfers may then be utilized to restore wrist and finger extension by transferring the flexor carpi ulnaris to the long finger extensors and the pronator teres to the extensor carpi radialis brevis tendon. If the palmaris longus is present, it may be transferred to the extensor pollicis longus for thumb extension. If it is not present, the flexor carpi ulnaris may also be utilized for thumb extension

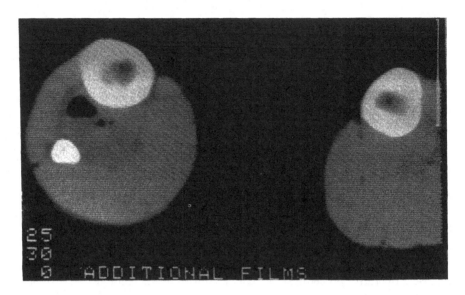

Fig. 2A. CAT scan which reveals extension into both anterior and posterior compartments secondary to previous biopsy.

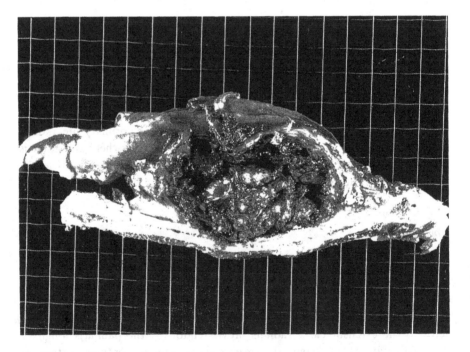

Fig. 2B. Since this was surgically converted to a IIb staging of the sarcoma, an amputation was necessary. The gross specimen reveals erosion into the fibula.

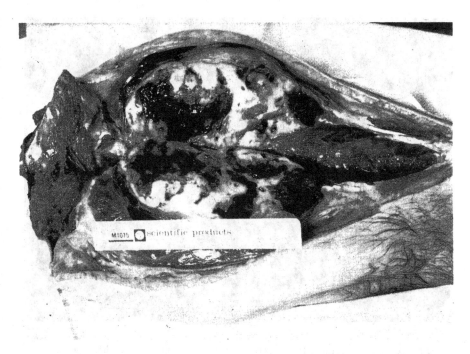

Fig. 3. A large IIb sarcoma of the buttock requiring a hemipelvectomy.

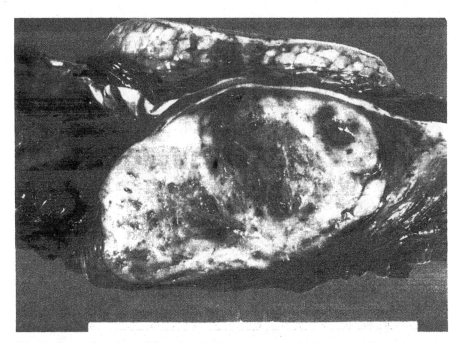

Fig. 4A. Resected specimen of the entire anterior compartment with the previous biopsy site excised in toto.

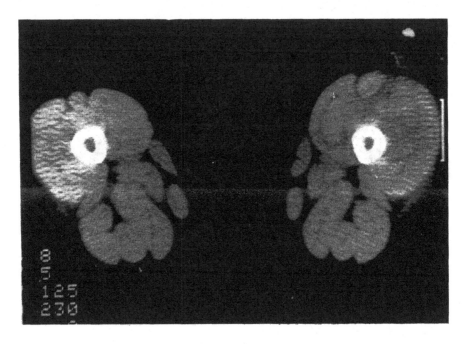

Fig. 4B. CAT scan illustrating a IIa sarcoma of the anterior compartment of the thigh.

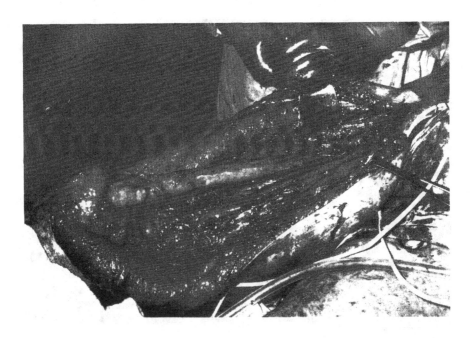

Fig. 4C. Entire anterior compartment has been resected preserving the knee joint as the sarcoma did not extend into the knee.

as well as finger extension. Other flexor tendons may be utilized for transfers such as the sublimis tendons. If diaphyseal segments of the radius and/or ulna must be resected, fibular bone grafts generally work well. If the wrist joint must be excised because of involvement, arthrodesis of the wrist functionally works well. If the elbow joint must be excised, depending upon the amount of bone stock left, bracing, arthrodesis, allograft, or arthroplasty (fascial or prosthetic) may be used, again, weighing the needs of the individual patient.

Anterior Compartment. The median and ulnar nerves lie together in the anterior compartment and if they must be sacrificed, junctional loss is so great that amputation would be preferred.

Arm

Posterior Compartment. The posterior compartment may be excised along with the radial nerve. Tendon transfers as described for posterior compartment of the forearm lesions may then be undertaken for hand function. Elbow function will remain quite good except for overhead work.

Anterior Compartment. Again, the median and ulnar nerves lie together in the anterior compartment and if they must be sacrificed, functional loss is so great that amputation would be preferred. If the sarcoma is in such a location that these structures can be preserved, the musculocutaneous nerve may be sacrificed with good functional results as the brachial radialis innervated by the radial nerve will provide for elbow flexion.

Shoulder

In sarcomas lying posterior to the scapula, the scapula may be removed with varying amounts of the proximal humerus as necessary preserving the rest of upper extremity function. If the sarcoma is anterior to the scapula, a portion of the chest cage with reconstruction of the chest is generally necessary. For sarcomas lying within the deltoid, resection of the entire deltoid from origin to insertion along with the proximal humerus may be undertaken. A fibular bone graft may then be utilized with an arthrodesis of the shoulder if the scapula can be preserved.

References

1. Albores-Saavedra J, Martin RG, Smith JL: Rhadomyosarcoma: A study of 35 cases. Ann Surg 157:186–197, 1963.
2. Adult Intergroup Soft-Tissue Sarcoma Committee: Recommendations for clinical protocol development and definition of therapeutic response for soft-tissue sarcomas. Cancer 46:796–800, 1980.
3. Baker HW: The surgical treatment of cancer. Cancer 43:787–789, 1979.
4. Bowden L, Booher RJ: The principles and techniques of resection of soft parts for sarcomas. Surgery 44:963–977, 1958.
5. Bowden L, Booher RJ: Surgical considerations in the treatment of sarcoma of the buttock. Cancer 6:89–99, 1953.
6. Broders AC, Hargrave R, Meyerding HW: Pathological features of soft tissue fibrosarcoma. With special reference to the grading of its malignancy. Surg Gynecol Obstet 69:267–280, 1939.
7. Cadman NL, Soule EH, Kelly PJ: Synovial sarcoma. An analysis of 134 tumors. Cancer 18:613–627, 1965.
8. Cantin J, McNeer GP, Chu FC, Booher RJ: The problem of local recurrence after treatment of soft tissue sarcoma. Ann Surg 168:47–53, 1968.
9. Castro EB, Hajdu SI, Fortner JG: Surgical therapy of fibrosarcoma of extremities. A re-appraisal. Arch Surg 107:284–286, 1973.
10. Changes in treating soft-tissue sarcomas. (Author not specified). Br Med J 2:562–563, 1979.
11. Clark RL Jr., Martin RG, White EC, Old JW: Clinical aspects of soft-tissue tumors. AMA Arch Surg 74:859–870, 1957.
12. Clay MG, Sandy JTM, Inman RJ: Short-term follow-up of surgically treated sarcomas. Am J Surg 141:537–538, 1981.
13. Eilber FR, Mirra JJ, Grant TT, Weisenburger T, Morton DL: Is amputation necessary for sarcomas? A seven-year experience with limb salvage. Ann Surg 192:431–438, 1980.
14. Enneking WF: Principles of musculoskeletal pathology. Gainesville, Florida: Storter Printing Co., 1977.
15. Enneking WF, Spanier SS, Malawer MM: The effect of the anatomic setting on the results of surgical procedures for soft parts sarcoma of the thigh. Cancer 47:1005–1022, 1981.
16. Enterline HT, Culberson JD, Rochlin DB, Brady LW: Liposarcoma. A clinical and pathological study of 53 cases. Cancer 13:932–950, 1960.
17. Enzinger FM, Shiraki M: Alveolar rhabdomyosarcoma. An analysis of 110 cases. Cancer 24:18–31, 1969.
18. Gerner RE, Moore GE, Pickren JW: Soft tissue sarcomas. Ann Surg 181:803–808, 1975.
19. Gilbert HA, Kagan AR, Winkley J: Management of soft-tissue sarcomas of the extremities. Surg Gynecol Obstet 39:1201–1217, 1977.
20. Krementz ET, Shaver JO: Behavior and treatment of soft tissue sarcomas. Ann Surg 157:770–784, 1963.
21. Lieberman Z, Ackerman LV: Principles in management of soft tissue sarcomas. A clinical and pathologic review of one hundred cases. Surgery 35:350–365, 1954.
22. Lindberg RD, Martin RG, Romsdahl MM, McMurtrey MJ: Conservative Surgery and Radiation Therapy for Soft Tissue Sarcomas. Chicago: Year Book Medical Publishers, 1977, pp 289–298.
23. Lunseth PA, Nelson CL: Longitudinal amputation for the treatment of soft tissue fibrosarcoma. Clin Orthop 109:147–151, 1975.
24. Martin RG, Butler JJ, Albores-Saavedra J: Soft tissue tumors: Surgical treatment and results. In: Tumors of Bone and Soft Tissue. Clinical Conference on Cancer, M.D. Anderson Hospital and Tumor Institute. Chicago: Year Book, 1965, pp 333–348.

25. Moberger G, Nilsonne U, Friberg S Jr.: Synovial sarcoma. histologic features and prognosis. Acta Orthop Scand Suppl 111:1–38, 1968.
26. Morton DL, Eilber FR, Townsend CM Jr., Grant TT, Mirra J, Weisenburger TH: Limb salvage from a multidisciplinary treatment approach for skeletal and soft tissue sarcomas of the extremity. Ann Surg 184:268–278, 1976.
27. Pack GT: End results in the treatment of sarcomata of the soft somatic tissues. J Bone Joint Surg 36-A:241–263, 1954.
28. Pritchard DJ, Soule EH, Taylor WF, Ivins JC: Fibrosarcoma – Clinicopathologic and statistical study of 199 tumors of the soft tissues of the extremities and trunk. Cancer 33:888–897, 1974.
29. Reszel PA, Soule EH, Coventry MB: Liposarcoma of the extremities and limb girdles. A study of two hundred twenty-two cases. J Bone Joint Surg 48-A:229–244, 1966.
30. Rosenberg SA, Webber BL, Chabner B, Chretien PB, Sears HF: Prospective randomized evaluation of the role of limb-sparing surgery, radiation therapy, and adjuvant chemoimmunotherapy in the treatment of adult soft-tissue sarcomas. Surgery 84:62–69, 1978.
31. Ryan JR, Baker LH, Benjamin RS: The natural history of metastatic synovial sarcoma (experience of the Southwest Oncology Group). Clin Orthop 164:253–256, 1982.
32. Sears HF, Hopson R, Inouye W, Rizzo T, Grotziner PJ: Analysis of staging and management of patients with sarcoma. A ten-year experience. Ann Surg 191:488–493, 1980.
33. Sears HF: Soft tissue sarcoma: A historical overview. Semin Oncol 8:129–132, June 1981.
34. Shieber W, Graham P: An experience with sarcomas of the soft tissues in adults. Surgery 52:295–298, 1962.
35. Shiu MH, Castro EB, Hajdu SI, Fortner JG: Surgical treatment of 297 soft tissue sarcomas of the lower extremity. Ann Surg 182:597–602, 1975.
36. Shiu MH, McCormack PM, Hajdu SI, Fortner JG: Surgical treatment of tendosynovial sarcoma. Cancer 43:889–897, 1979.
37. Simon MA: Management of adult soft-tissue sarcomas of the extremities. Surg Ann 11:363–402, 1979.
38. Simon MA, Enneking WF: The management of soft-tissue sarcomas of the extremities. J Bone Joint Surg 58-A:317–327, 1976.
39. Soule EH, Enriquez P: Atypical fibrous histiocytoma, malignant fibrous histiocytoma, malignant histiocytoma, and epithelioid sarcoma. A comparative study of 65 tumors. Cancer 30:128–143, 1972.
40. Storm FK, Eilber FR, Mirra J, Morton DL: Neurofibrosarcoma. Cancer 45:126–129, 1980.
41. Stout AP: Liposarcomas. The malignant tumor of lipoblasts. Ann Surg 119:86–107, 1944.
42. Stout AP: Fibrosarcoma. The malignant tumor of fibroblasts. Cancer 1:30–63, 1948.
43. Suit HD, Russell WO, Martin RG: Sarcoma of soft tissue: Clinical and histopathologic parameters and response to treatment. Cancer 35:1478–1483, 1975.
44. Suit HD, Russell WO, Martin RG: Management of patients with sarcoma of soft tissue in an extremity. Cancer 31:1247–1255, 1973.
45. Suit HD, Russell WO: Soft part tumors. Cancer 39:830–836, 1977.
46. Suit HD, Proppe KH, Mankin HJ, Woods WC: Preoperative radiation therapy for sarcoma of soft tissue. Cancer 47:2269–2274, 1981.
47. Thompson DE, Frost HM, Hendrick JW, Horn RC Jr.: Soft tissue sarcomas involving the extremities and the limb girdles: A review. South Med J 64:33–44, 1971.
48. van der Werf-Messing B, van Unnik JAM: Fibrosarcoma of the soft tissues. A clinicopathologic study. Cancer 18:1113–1123, 1965.
49. Wanebo HJ, Shah J, Knapper W, Hajdu S, Booher R: Reappraisal of surgical management of sarcoma of the buttock. Cancer 31:97–104, 1973.

5. Cyto Reduction for Soft Tissue Sarcomas

CHARLES E. LUCAS and ANNA M. LEDGERWOOD

Eradication of all malignant disease is the uniform objective of therapy. Such eradication usually is achieved by surgical excision, whereas, in some instances a tumor may be best treated by chemotherapy, radiation therapy, or some combination of all three. Surgical excision, alone, as a definitive treatment of many gastrointestinal carcinomas yields a cure when the disease is diagnosed prior to extension though the gut wall and when adequate margins beyond the gross tumor are included in the resected specimen. This type of resection allows for a three-dimensional or circumferential excision of both tumor and surrounding tumor free tissues. Surgical excision of other tumors such as the papillary adenocarcinomas of the thyroid will be associated with long-term free interval even through a wide margin of tumor free tissue is not incorporated with the resected specimen; long-term thyroid replacement therapy facilitates suppression of subsequent tumor growth. Other tumors such as embryonal cell sarcomas in males and choriocarcinoma in females may be most effectively treated with chemotherapy with surgical excision being used primarily for diagnosis, cyto reduction and stem cell analysis.

The therapeutic challenges related to soft tissue sarcomas, especially those in the retroperitoneal space, require a unique approach which embodies many of the principles outlined above but with a special selective emphasis. In contrast to the soft tissue sarcomas of the extremity which may be eradicated for cure by wide excision including four quarter or hind quarter amputation or by wide excision plus chemotherapy, the retroperitoneal soft tissue sarcomas seldom are accessible to wide excision with disease free margins. The retroperitoneal space is an undesirable site for sarcomatous growth since the early symptoms are often nonspecific as continued growth does not interfere with specific organ function until the tumor has reached large proportions. All too frequently a large bulky tumor is present by the time a specific diagnosis is suspected [3, 6]. Once the diagnosis is confirmed, extension to adjacent structures is the rule. This extension often involves the paravertebral muscles, especially, the psoas muscles, the kidney, adrenal gland, posterior parieties, peritoneum, transversalis muscle and fascia, and ipsilateral hemidiaphragm; other structures such as the ipsilateral

Baker, L.H. (ed.), Soft Tissue Sarcomas. ISBN 0-89838-584-9
© *1983 Martinus Nijhoff Publishers, Boston/The Hague/Dordrecht/Lancaster. Printed in the Netherlands.*

ureter, ipsilateral great vessels, and ipsilateral hollow viscera may be compromised by compression or invasion from the unrelenting expansion of such an ubiquitous malignant mass. Finally, these masses have no respect for anatomic regions and may extend up into the thorax or down into the pelvis.

For many reasons the technical challenges of surgical extirpation of such tumors are overwhelming. Firstly, the technical armamentarium of most surgeons does not include well defined operative approaches to large retroperitoneal tumors. These tumors which often invest multiple organ systems, by definition, cross surgical specialty jurisdictions. Consequently, the general surgical skills of dealing with hollow viscera provide little help in the extraction of that portion of tumor which involves the genital urinary system, major vessels, hemidiaphragm, or chest wall. Secondly, major technical problems revolve around the extent of tumor excision. Whereas one can readily achieve a wide circumferential excision of a hollow visceral tumor through an anterior approach or of a selected adrenal tumor by way of a posterior approach, the large retroperitoneal soft tissue sarcoma requires a combined anterior-posterior or anterior-lateral approach in order to provide access to multiple anatomic regions. Attempts to employ incisions which are designed specifically for an anterior or a posterior problem will lead to inadequate tumor exposure which in turn increases the likelihood of significant bleeding consequent to dissection in regions which are not properly exposed. The results of such endeavors lead to life-threatening hemorrhage, incomplete excision of the tumor, and increased postoperative morbidity and mortality related to the homeostatic sequela of hemorrhagic shock. Singular frustrating experiences by multiple surgeons facilitate the evolution of a collective view that such tumors are to be feared, shunned, and referred to the Oncology Service after the careful obtainment of sufficient tissue for diagnosis and stem cell analysis. Unfortunately, a therapeutic view is promulgated that such tumors must be approached with great trepidation and this surgical affect is indirectly abetted in many surgical training programs. Consequently, the definitive care of such tumors has fallen into the hands of the radiotherapist and oncologist who have embarked upon several well defined protocols of chemotherapy and/or radiation therapy. Although such regimens have provided excellent information concerning tumor response to several therapeutic agents, the effects of these treatments are limited. Recurrence with further local extensions, distant spread, and finally death from disease are the rule. Although the initial response to chemotherapy may be encouraging, the chemotherapeutic agents often are totally unresponsive, produce only a limited response resulting in partial remission, or connot be reused because of organ toxicity in those patients who develop recurrence after a complete remission [1, 9, 10].

During the past decade a more aggressive surgical approach to these retroperitoneal tumors has evolved. Greater surgical fortitude has resulted in the excision of many retroperitoneal sarcomas which cross organ system boundaries and anatomic regions. These excisions, however, are not curative since the margins of resection, by definition, are adjacent to the mass and the operator leaves residual microscopic tumor even though all gross tumor has been excised. Although an excellent complete remission may be obtained by this modality, recurrences are the rule and eventually lead to the patients demise. The objectives of the present report are to outline, from a surgical prospective, a reasonable approach to these soft tissue retroperitoneal sarcomas. This approach calls for surgical cyto reduction of either the primary sarcoma or the metastatic sarcoma involving non-adjacent anatomic sites such as the lungs and liver. Theoretically, cyto reduction by surgical excision of all gross tumor combined with radiation therapy and chemotherapy should enhance the time of complete remission and partial remission or, in selected instances, bring about a permanent cure. The emphasis, herein, is threefold, namely, (1) the primary excision of a retroperitoneal soft tissue sarcoma, (2) the excision of a metastatic tumor as part of cyto reduction, and (3) the palliative excision of metastatic tumor in patients with non-curable disease in order to enhance comfort and assist further palliative therapy through information obtained by stem cell analysis.

Historical Notes

Recent advances in the use of multiple drug therapy have established a foundation upon which subsequent progress can be made. These advances, in particular, have revolved around Adriamycin as a backbone of therapy for soft tissue sarcoma [5]. Using multiple drug therapy, Buchanan and Yap reported an 18% complete remission rate and a 49% combined complete plus partial remission rate in those patients with soft tissue sarcoma being treated by the combination of Cy VADIC (Cyclophosphamide, Vincristine, Adriamycin, Dimethyl Triazeno Imidazole Carboxamide) [1, 10]. Furthermore, they noted that a complete remission obtained by chemotherapy is as long as a complete remission obtained by the combination of chemotherapy and operative excision of the soft tissue sarcoma [1]. Unfortunately, Adriamycin, which is the mainstay for long-term therapy of these tumors, is cardiotoxic when given over repeated dosages so that long therapy is severely compromised when a patient has recieved the maximum safe level of Adriamycin. Although Buchanan and Yap were able to show that Adriamycin is much less toxic when given by way of a continuous infusion, cardiotoxicity is still a major problem if more than 12–18 courses of chemotherapy are given [1].

Based upon the limitations of chemotherapy, particularly Adriamycin therapy, a reasonable approach for enhancing the incidence of complete remission includes the resection of all gross tumor after three consecutive doses of chemotherapy followed by the re-institution of chemotherapy during the postoperative period for an undetermined time, possibly for 18 months. Benjamin and Yap reported on a group of 50 patients ranging in age from 16 to 75 years with an average of 42 years who were entered into a prospective study in which this type of approach was implemented [1]. Twenty-six or 52% of these patients had distant metastases located primarily in the lungs, whereas the remaining patients had far advanced local disease from a bulky expanding soft tissue sarcoma. The most frequent cell type was a malignant fibrous histiocytoma (13 patients) followed by neurogenic sarcoma (6 patients), angiosarcoma (5 patients), leiomyosarcoma (5 patients) and unclassified sarcomas (5 patients) [1, 2, 4, 7]. During the initial course of preoperative chemotherapy, seven patients (14%) went into a complete remission, whereas 20 patients (40%) had a partial remission as defined by 50% reduction in tumor size. At the same time four of the patients had minor decrease in tumor size; nine patients had no change in tumor size, whereas the tumor grew more than 20% during the period of chemotherapy in 10 patients (20%). Significantly, none of the patients with far advanced local disease had a complete remission during this period of preoperative chemotherapy. This lack of complete remission in this large group of patients indicates the futility of chemotherapy alone in patients with massive bulky soft tissue sarcomas. The response to both chemotherapy plus operative cyto reduction was encouraging. There were 25 patients with residual tumor who underwent operative cyto reduction. Complete reduction of all gross tumor remaining after the preoperative chemotherapy was accomplished in 15 patients (60% of those undergoing operative cyto reduction) all of whom had a complete remission. An additional nine patients had minimal gross disease left behind and they had a partial remission. The combination of chemotherapy alone or chemotherapy followed by operative cyto reduction of residual tumor, therefore, was associated with a complete remission in 22 of the 50 patients, whereas 37 of the 50 patients had either a complete remission or a partial remission. More significantly the complete remission in this combined group of patients lasted for an average of 25 months and 75% of patients with complete remission were still alive at 22 months following the initiation of therapy [1].

The significant improvement with this combined form of therapy raises the question as to whether some of these soft tissue sarcomas might not be cured by the combination of operative cyto reduction and chemotherapy. Theoretically, the ability of the chemotherapeutic agents to attack a minute number of residual malignant cells left along the border of the resected specimen should enhance the likelihood for cure. Since a cure may result from operative cyto reduction of all gross tumor when used in conjunction with chemotherapy, the risk/benefit ratio of performing excessive surgical excision in the face of major technical impediments is shifted in favor of excision for possible cure. Some of the principles related to this type of therapy including the technical and physiologic problems associated with combined surgery and chemotherapy are well illustrated by the following case report.

Case Report #1

This 77-year-old female first presented to another hospital with signs and symptoms suggesting acute intestinal obstruction. Following initial hydration and nasogastric decompression she was prepared for operative intervention at which time a large retroperitoneal mass was encountered. This mass was thought to involve the pancreas and part of the duodenum; only an incisional biopsy with partial resection was accomplished in the face of significant bleeding. During the post operative period a necrotic brownish drainage exuded from a left upper quadrant drain site which had been left adjacent to the site of partial tumor resection. Gradually, gastrointestinal function returned and she was discharged and referred to the Oncology Service in July, 1981.

A fistulagram through the drain at this time showed cutaneous communication with a large necrotic mass located throughout most of the left retroperi-

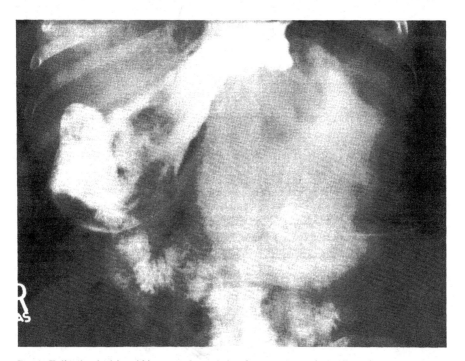

Fig. 1. Following incisional biopsy performed elsewhere persistent drainage of the necrotic tumor center required prolonged dressing change but was confirmed by a sinus tract injection to be separate from the bowel.

toneal space with extension to the left lobe of the liver and probable extension to left sided hollow viscera (Fig. 1). Chemotherapy with Adriamycin and Dimethyl Triazeno Imidazol Carboxamide was initiated. Subsequent courses of therapy with the same two agents were given in August and September of 1981. Despite the chemotherapy, the subjective response was unremarkable and the tumor continued to expand. Discussion regarding excisional therapy took place at this time but in view of the risk involved with such excision and because the patient had reasonable restoration of gastrointestinal function, it was decided to defer surgery until a date when the patient was more symptomatic.

Seven months later, by April, 1982, the patient noted further growth of this massive tumor which was now pushing the left rib cage and left upper quadrant anteriorly and all of the intra-abdominal viscera to the right so that the 'right of domain' of the hollow viscera was being challenged (Fig. 2). After the technical hazards of surgical intervention were explained to the patient and her relatives, preparations for operative intervention were made. Roentgenographic evaluation at this time showed that the tumor caused marked right-sided deviation of the stomach and small bowel (Fig. 3), inferior displacement of the colon (Fig.

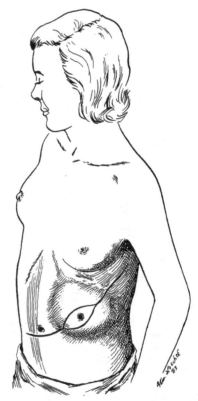

Fig. 2. Prior to definitive resection the huge mass caused marked deviation of the left lower chest wall and the whole left side of the abdomen with extension across the midline.

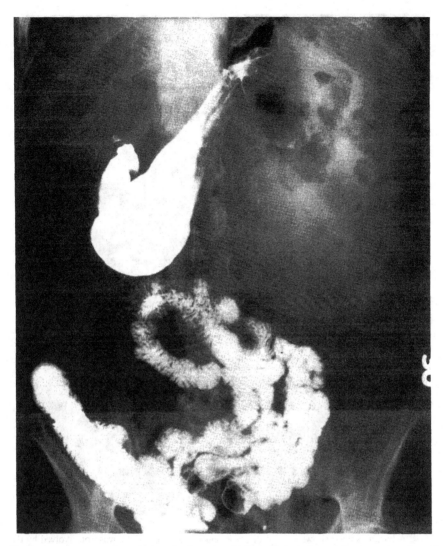

Fig. 3. An upper gastrointestinal study shows marked lateral deviation of the stomach and small bowel and irregularity along the greater curvature of the stomach which had to be resected because of direct extension of the tumor.

4), and probable local invasion or crowding of adjacent organ such as the left hemidiaphragm, abdominal wall, spleen, pancreas, and kidney as viewed on the CAT scan (Fig. 5).

The initial incision was made along the left ninth rib and extended in an oblique manner down to just below the umbilicus where the incision was curved in a transverse manner to the right and extended to the right anterior-axillary line to provide access to the tumor extension on the right side of both the in-

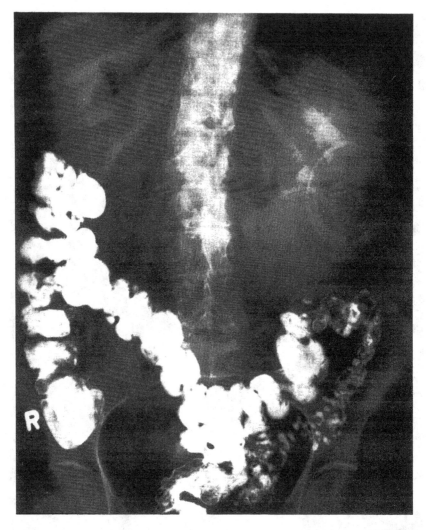

Fig. 4. A barium enema shows inferior displacement of the colon which was not involved by the tumor although the mesentary of the colon had to be resected because of direct invasion.

traperitoneal and retroperitoneal cavities (Fig. 5). This incision allowed for maximal exposure of the left lower thorax, left retroperitoneum, most intra-abdominal contents, and the left pelvic structures. That portion of the tumor which had fistulized through the skin and had invaded full-thickness abdominal wall was included within an island of skin and full-thickness abdominal wall which was included with the initial incision. Once the outer margins of the tumor were encountered, meticulous dissection from the surrounding structures to which it was attached with multiple small vessels was required to maintain

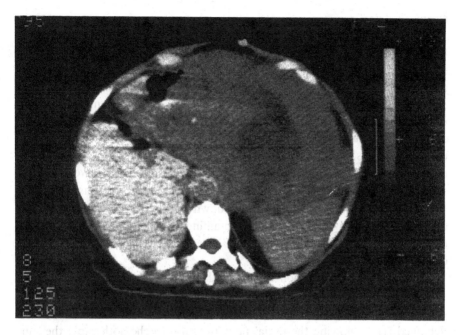

Fig. 5. The CAT scan shows evidence of multiple involvement and compression of the normal intraperitoneal vescera to the point that the 'right of domain' was threatened.

careful hemostasis by means of electrocoagulation and suture ligature. By gradually encompassing the tumor in this manner, the mass could be gradually freed-up to those sites where dense adhesions or invasion of adjacent structures required resection of these structures with the total mass. Those structures which had to be included with the resection were a portion of the left hemidiaphragm, a portion of the greater curvature of the stomach, a segment of the left lobe of the liver, the spleen, part of the distal pancreas, and the mesentary to a segment of small bowel and the left colon. Vascular integrity to the left colon was preserved by means of the marginal artery of Drummond. The operative procedure lasted approximately eight hours and, post-operatively, the patient was maintained on a volume ventilator until the next morning when extubation was successfully achieved. Her subsequent postoperative course was uneventful. The final pathological diagnosis was probable fibrosarcoma with suggestive features of a malignant fibrous histiocytoma. Nineteen months following surgical excision, the patient continues to be in complete remission.

Comment

Many of the features in the above presentation highlight the difficulties with early diagnosis for these tumors. The symptoms related to the gastrointestinal tract on the initial admission were really reflective of a large bulky mass causing compression of hollow viscera rather than intrinsic obstruction. The need to perform emergency surgery on a presumptive diagnosis of bowel obstruction compromised the preoperative preparation in terms of diagnosis, patient preparation and also surgeon preparation. The initial horizontal transperitoneal incision compromised the surgeon's ability to define, intraoperatively, the full extent of this bulky mass and led to futile attempts to resect this massive tumor, the true extent of which was not fully known at this original procedure. The consequent decision to 'backout' after obtaining sufficient tissue for biopsy and decompressing the central liquefaction reflected good judgement in this difficult circumstance.

The subsequent poor response to chemotherapy is typical for these tumors in which the vast bulk has been left behind. Buchanan and Yap reported no complete remissions when the major portion of the tumor could not be surgically debulked [1]. Following the initial poor response to chemotherapy, the subsequent delay in surgical debulking reflected a combination of events including patient fear that excision of this tumor would likely cause intraoperative exsanguination as so indicated by her initial surgeon. Once the tumor had reached significantly larger proportions, the symptoms of organ compression were such that the patient was willing to risk death rather than continue to live in this compromised matter. This sequence of events is common for these massive tumors. Just as common is the surgical decision to observe rather than re-operate.

Once the decision is made to attempt resection of these massive tumors, a very complete preoperative evaluation is essential to provide maximum knowledge as to the intraoperative challenges which will be encountered. The CAT scan is the single most valuable test for determining the soft tissue extensions of these bulky retroperitoneal masses [8]. Once resection is engaged upon, however, precise knowledge of the vascular extension must be accomplished by means of aortography and inferior venacavography, the latter being obtained in order to determine whether ligation or graft interposition may be required at the time of resection [3, 6]. Pylography and retrograde ureterography are essential to determine whether excision of the ipsilateral kidney and ureter may also be needed. An extensive bowel prep is essential not only to reduce the bacterial content within the bowel in preparation for possible resection but also to eliminate all gas which might cause bowel distension and interfere with safe bowel resection, if necessary. The bowel prep should be combined with the systemic administration of appropriate antibiotics. Once these preparations have been made, the likelihood for a successful complete excision of all gross tumor is enhanced and the subsequent good result as seen herein may be expected. During the operative resection, the placement of hemoclips in order to assist in subsequent radiation therapy is probably not warranted in that the hemoclips will diminish the precision of subsequent CAT scans which must be obtained as part of the follow-up examination. After a patient has obtained a complete remission by this modality subsequent chemotherapy as outlined above will enhance the prolongation of this complete remission and will, possibly, lead to cure. The role of the second look operation as a postoperative diagnostic and therapeutic modality is diminished by the enhanced diagnostic capabilities of the CAT scan which will identify recurrent tumor with just about the same accuracy as an operative second look procedure [3, 8]. Recurrent tumor once suspected, however, should be approached with the same aggressiveness as the original tumor using appropriate combination of operative excision and, if possible, additional chemotherapy.

Problems with Metastatic tumors

Pulmonary Metastasis

Although some patients with massive soft tissue sarcomas have local spread to multiple organs which must be resected as part of the original tumor, other patients present with distant metastasis most commonly to the liver and/or the lung. When the original tumor is under control, recent data suggest that an aggressive approach to both the pulmonary and liver metastatic lesions is appropriate. Most clinical information regarding this approach has been obtained in the treatment of pulmonary metastasis which, when performed in conjunction with appropriate radiation therapy and chemotherapy, may result in a significant complete remission or partial remission and in some instances apparent cure. Some of the beneficial aspects of this aggressive approach as it relates to excision of pulmonary metastasis are outlined in the following case report.

Case Report #2

This 57-year-old physician first presented in 1978 with a left intrascapular mass measuring approximately two centimeters in diameter. Local excision of this tumor was performed and the histologic diagnosis was compatible with fibrosarcoma. Postoperative radiation therapy and chemotherapy were subsequently employed. Local recurrence of the tumor in July, 1979 was treated by wider local resection after which the patient was again started on radiation therapy. Since the margins of resection showed residual tumors, an even wider local excision was performed in August, 1979 followed by more raddition therapy.

Following an uneventful asymptomatic six month interval, a follow-up chest x-ray revealed two nodules in the right lung which were considered to be metastatic lesions. Following a complete evaluation of these lesions, a right thoracotomy was perfomed and the two nodules, a 5 mm nodule in the right upper lobe and an 8 mm nodule in the right lower lobe, were removed by a generous wedge resection from each lobe. During this admission a suspected nodule in the left lung was shown by CAT scan to be a non-existant. Following this operative procedure the patient had an asymptomatic interval of 21 months when he represented with two masses along the left chest wall in proximity to the previous local exicisions.

Following complete evaluation for more distant tumor, a local excision of the soft tissues overlying the chest wall including the entire left latissimus dorsi muscle was accomplished and split-thickness skin grafts were placed over that portion of the wound which could not be approximated primarily. The resected recurrent tumor was interpreted to be a malignant fibrous histiocytoma and the margins of resection were again clear. The postoperative course was complicated by some loss of the split-thickness skin graft but the wound subsequently healed by second intent and the patient returned to a normal activity which included intensive rehabilitation to the point where he was able to run in the local marathons.

This procedure was followed by another 12 months of complete remission. A follow-up chest x-ray in November, 1982 showed a recurrent nodule in the right upper lobe (Fig. 6). Following a negative work-up for other disease, a thoracotomy was performed through the same right posterior-lateral incision and a right upper lobectomy was accomplished for a 3 × 5 cm metastatic lesion in the right upper lobe. Although the technical aspects of the operation were difficult because of adhesions from the prior thoracotomy, the patient had an uncomplicated postoperative course and has entered into another phase of complete remission.

Comment

The sequence of events occurring in this patient highlight many features in patients with local soft tissue sarcoma which may require multiple procedures for control of the primary site and be associated with recurrent metastatic lesions to the lung. The metastatic lesions are best treated by aggressive local excision in combination with adjuvant chemotherapy and/or radiation therapy. Excisional cyto reduction allows for more effective adjuvant therapy and, when possible, should include all metastatic disease to enhance the chances for complete remission. When nodules are noted in both lung fields, all nodules should be removed,

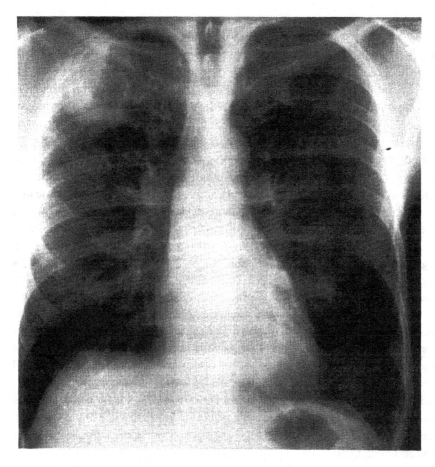

Fig. 6. Chest x-ray shows recurrent right upper lobe metastasis which was resected through a second right thoracotomy.

preferably, at the same operative procedure. The surgical approach to pulmonary metastatic nodules confined to one lung may be best removed by the classic posterior-lateral thoracotomy. When lesions are located in both lung fields, the operative approach may consist of bilateral small thoracotomies when the lesions are not readily accessible to a single incision. When bilateral lesions are located anteriorly in both lung fields, they may be excised through a median sternotomy. Alternatively, the lesion may be excised by a transverse thoracotomy extending across the sternum into both thoraces. Regardless of the technical approach, the underlying objective ahould be complete removal of all metastatic lesions to increase the incidence and the duration of complete remission.

Liver Metastasis

Another common site for distant metastases from the soft tissue sarcomas is the liver. Theoretically, the same principles of treatment apply, namely, resection of all metastatic disease in patients in whom such an operative insult is thought to be compatible with survival and in whom the non-resected liver parenchyma will support life. Normally, about 30% of the liver must be preserved to maintain vital liver function.

Important technical considerations arise when hepatic resection of metastatic nodules is being planned. The vascularity of the liver is more complex than the pulmonary vascularity with the result that multiple resections of liver tissue may be associated with more hemorrhage and greater overall risk to the patient. The liver has a dual blood supply from both the hepatic artery and the portal vein. Precise identification of the hepatic artery distribution is essential in view of the high incidence of arterial anatomic anomalies. The arterial anomalies of the hepatic arterial system have been well defined (Fig. 7). When the vascular anomaly is such that not all of the hepatic branches come from the celiac axis, additional views of the superior mesenteric artery distribution will identify the most frequent anomaly, whereby the right hepatic artery arises from the superior mesenteric artery. Knowledge of the hepatic venous anatomy, both lobar and segmental, permits a rational and safe resection of intrahepatic nodules (Fig. 8). The extent of liver resection will also be determined by the relationship between a metastatic nodule and the boundaries of the various segments (Fig. 9). A concise knowledge of the hepatic segmental anatomy facilitates this safe and appropriate resection of metastatic nodules while preserving the maximal amount of uninvolved parenchyma.

The anatomic approach for such resections can be accomplished by means of a midline laparotomy with cephlad extension as a median sternotomy. This permits complete exposure to both lobes of the liver when the diaphragm is divided in its median plane. Likewise, access to all of the hepatic veins is enhanced by this incision. Alternatively, an oblique incision extending along the bed of the right eight or ninth rib and carried in a caudad direction along the same plane to the left side of the umbilicus permits wide access to those lesions which are located along the dome of the right lobe in proximity to the bare surface of the liver and to the right heptatic vein. The key to successful resection is wide and thorough exposure of the liver and its adjacent organs. The specifics regarding the actual resection of metastatic lesions have been described elsewhere; emphasis however, should be placed on the local excision or wedge resection of intrahepatic nodules in lieu of anatomic lobextomy whenever disease free margins can be accomplished by the lesser resection. Although, the wedge resection through non-anatomic planes requires a more fastidious control of cross-linking vessels and liver suture hemostasis of oozing parenchyma (Fig. 10), this procedure permits

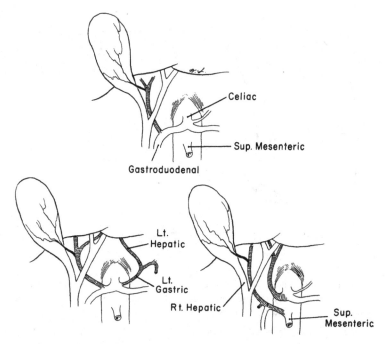

Fig. 7. Prior to resection of hepatic metastasis, clear delineation of normal and abnormal hepatic arterial anatomy is required; the most common arterial anatomy is shown, whereby the right hepatic artery arises from the superior mesenteric artery.

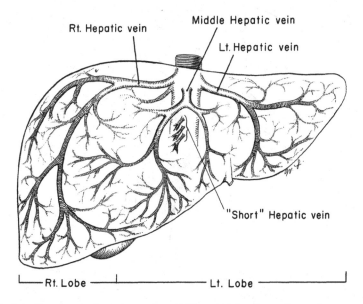

Fig. 8. The hepatic venous anatomy does not parallel the arterial anatomy; the most common venous drainage is shown here.

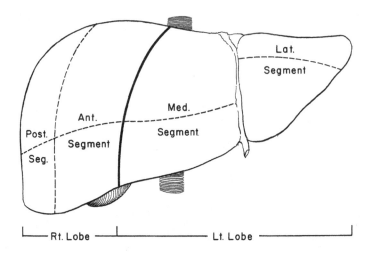

Fig. 9. Wedge resection of multiple metastatic nodules is usually the preferred treatment although larger metastatic lesions may require segmentectomy or lobectomy; a thorough knowledge of parenchymal anatomy as show here is essential.

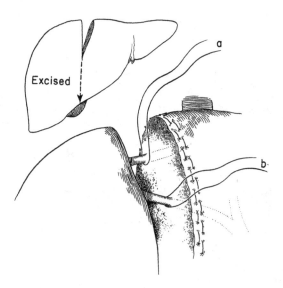

Fig. 10. During partial hepatic resection, careful hemostasis with the combination of individual ligation of cross-linking vessels plus liver suture of oozing parenchyma is essential.

the maximal preservation of uninvolved parenchyma. When the major portion of a lobe is involved, the simplest and most effective way to provide for a safe cyto reduction is formal lobectomy.

Resection of Metastatic Disease for Palliation

Many patients have diffuse disease which is beyond the point at which surgical cure or even partial remission can be affected. Soft tissue sarcomas which have advanced beyond the point of even partial remission tend to metastasize in a rather diffuse manner. Commonly such patients will present with cutaneous or subcutaneous metastatic nodules which produce a myriad of symptoms such as pain, tenderness, overlying necrosis with bleeding and foul odor, and erosion into adjacent bony structures particularly the skull. Although radiation therapy may reduce some of the osseous problems with these metastatic nodules, the vast majority of these metastatic nodules are best treated by local excision. Such excision provides tremendous palliation in terms of comfort and in terms of the patients psychological status. This is particularly true when the metastatic lesions are located in genital areas, areas of obvious exposure to friends, and in the scalp. Local excision of these lesions must often be accomplished with local anesthesia since metastatic disease in other sites such as the liver and lung precludes safe general anesthesia. Besides enhancing patient comfort, these excised nodules can also be used for stem cell analysis in order to increase the likelihood of response to additional chemotherapy.

References

1. Benjamin RS, Yap B: Infusion chemotherapy for soft tissue sarcomas. Chapter 8, this volume.
2. Braasch JW, Mon AB: Primary retroperitoneal tumors. Surg Clin North Am 47:663–78, 1967.
3. Bryant RL, Stevenson DR, Hunton DW, et al.: Primary malignant retroperitoneal tumors. Am J Surg 144:647–49, 1982.
4. Gill W, Carter DC, Durie B: Retroperitoneal tumors. J R Coll Surg Edinburgh 15:213–21, 1950.
5. Gottlieb JA, Baker LH, O'Bryan RM, et al.: Adriamycin used alone and in combination for soft tissue and bony sarcomas. Cancer Chemother Rep 6:271–82, 1975.
6. Moore S, Aldrete J: Primary retroperitoneal sarcomas: the role of surgical treatment. Am J Surg 142:358–61, 1981.
7. Pack GT, Tabah EJ: Collective review: primary retroperitoneal tumors, study of 120 cases. Int Abstr Surg 99:209–31, 313–41, 1954.
8. Stephens DW, Sheedy PF, Hattery RR, et al.: Diagnosis and evaluation of retroperitoneal tumors by computerized tomography. Am J Radiol 129:395–402, 1977.
9. Storm FK, Eiber FR, Mirra J, et al.: Retroperitoneal sarcomas: a reappraisal of treatment. J Surg Oncol 17:1–7, 1981.
10. Yap BS, Sinkovics JG, Benjamin RS, et al.: Survival and relapse patterns of complete responders in adults with advanced soft tissue sarcomas. Proc Am Soc Clin Oncol 20:352, 1979.

6. Adjuvant Chemotherapy of Adult Soft Tissue Sarcomas

STEVEN A. ROSENBERG

Introduction

Though many single agents and combination chemotherapy regimens have been developed with excellent activity against metastatic soft tissue sarcomas in the adult, few well designed clinical trials have been conducted utilizing chemotherapy as a postoperative adjuvant in the treatment of adults with soft tissue sarcomas [1].

Several factors have combined to make the study of adjuvant chemotherapy in adult soft tissue sarcomas difficult. The infrequent incidence of this tumor has made it difficult for any single group to accrue enough cases to meaningfully conduct a clinical trial in a reasonable period of time. Further, the heterogeneity of soft tissue sarcomas has also discouraged the conduct of clinical trials in this disease. Over 50 individual diagnoses form the constellation of diseases known as soft tissue sarcomas. In addition these diseases are not confined to an individual anatomic structure such as is the case for many other tumors. Diversity of diagnoses and locations have served to make each patient with soft tissue sarcoma appear somewhat unique and difficult to group with other patients in the same disease category.

The diagnosis and grading of soft tissue sarcomas represents one of the most difficult areas of modern oncologic pathology [2, 3]. Exact criteria for establishing the histologic cell of origin and for establishing the grade of individual sarcomas are not consistent among pathologists and disagreement in diagnoses and grading are frequent. New diagnoses have become popular in recent years that were not in common use previously and this has served to complicate comparison of current clinical trials with previously reported results [3].

Recent advances in understanding the natural biology of soft tissue sarcomas in the adult have, however, made it possible to overcome many of the problems surrounding the design of clinical trials in this disease. With the exception of selected rare diagnoses it has become apparent in recent years that the natural history and clinical course of patients with similar histologic grades of soft tissue sarcoma are similar for virtually all histologic types [1]. The most important

Baker, L.H. (ed.), Soft Tissue Sarcomas. ISBN 0-89838-584-9
© *1983 Martinus Nijhoff Publishers, Boston/The Hague/Dordrecht/Lancaster. Printed in the Netherlands.*

prognostic feature, by far, in patients with soft tissue sarcomas is the histologic grade of the lesion. For lesions of Grade III (most undifferentiated) soft tissue sarcomas will behave similarly regardless of histologic type. By grading sarcomas it has thus become possible to categorize these diagnoses into common groups that lend themselves to stratification in clinical trials.

Another important stratification criteria to consider is the location of the lesion. Patients with lesions of the extremities should be considered separately from patients with lesions of the head, neck and trunk. This division is arbitrary and further subdivisions are necessary since proximal extremity lesions are somewhat more difficult to treat than distal extremity lesions. In addition, lesions of the head, neck and trunk often pose formidable problems in achieving local control not seen in lesions in other locations. Studies of adjuvant chemotherapy of patients with soft tissue sarcomas must take these major prognostic variables into account to assure that patient groups are comparable.

When these criteria are accounted for it is possible to predict with some accuracy the course of patients with adult soft tissue sarcomas. A review of the five year survival from several reported series is presented in Table 1 [4–11]. In virtually all reported series five year survival of adult patients with soft tissue sarcomas is about 40%. In virtually all series, approximately 80% of patients who recur, recur within the first two years after initial definitive treatment [12–14]. This rapid rate of recurrence enables one to evaluate adjuvant therapy in a shorter period of time than for many other solid tumors.

Though the diagnosis of patients with soft tissue sarcomas is considered in detail elsewhere in this book, one factor should be emphasized as it relates to adjuvant studies. Soft tissue sarcomas metastasize virtually exclusively to the lung during the initial portions of their natural history. It is thus of crucial importance to study the lung for evidence of metastases prior to admitting patients into adjuvant trials if comparable groups of well-defined patients are to be studied. Approximately 10% of adult patients with soft tissue sarcomas present for the first time with evidence of pulmonary metastases on standard chest x-ray [5, 12]. All patients entering adjuvant trials should be studied with full lung tomography. Though many groups also use computed axial tomography to examine the lungs for evidence of metastatic disease we have found that over 75% of all lesions seen on computed tomographic studies of the lungs that are not seen on full lung tomograms represent benign lesions when evaluated at thoracotomy [15].

Only two groups have studied, in well controlled clinical trials, the efficacy of adjuvant chemotherapy in adult patients with soft tissue sarcomas. In this chapter the studies of these two groups will be reviewed in detail.

Adjuvant Chemotherapy with VACAR

Design of the Trial

From October, 1973 to September, 1976 59 patients at the M.D. Anderson Hospital with soft tissue sarcomas of the head, neck, trunk and extremities were entered into a prospective trial of the efficacy of adjuvant chemotherapy in addition to surgery and postoperative irradiation [16]. Of the 59 patients, 12 had lesions in the head and neck and abdomen and all of these patients received adjuvant chemotherapy. Of the remaining 47 patients with primary lesions of the trunk and extremities, 27 were randomized to receive chemotherapy and 20 were randomized to receive no chemotherapy. To achieve local control all patients received local surgical excision and postoperative irradiation. Details of the radiation technique have been published. In brief, a tumor dose of 6500 rads was given in 6–1/2 weeks, using a shrinking field after 5000 rads. For lesions in the abdomen the dose ranged from 5000 rads in five weeks to 5500 rads in 5–1/2 weeks.

Patients randomized to receive chemotherapy received the VACAR regimen. This consisted of:

1. Vincristine – 1.5 mg/m^2 (top dose limit 2 mg/dose) i.v. on day 1. Day 1 of the chemotherapy coincided with day 1 of the radiotherapy. Vincristine was continued weekly for 9 weeks, and then on day 1 of each chemotherapy cycle.
2. Adriamycin – 60 mg/m^2 i.v. on day 2 and repeated every 4 weeks for 7 doses (total dose limit 420 mg/m^2).
3. Cyclophosphamide – 200 mg/m^2 orally on days 3, 4, and 5 of each cycle. Cyclophosphamide was repeated every 4 weeks with Adriamycin and every 8

Table 1. Soft tissue sarcomas: 5-year survival.

Group	Number of patients	Survival (%)	
		5-year	10-year
Task Force, AJC	1,215	41	30
Surgery Branch, NCI (before 1975)	66	48	44
Gerner *et al.*	155	50	26
Shieber *et al.*	125	27	22
Martin *et al.*	183	40	–
Pack *et al.*	717	39	–
Hare *et al.*	200	39	–
Shiu *et al.*	297	55	41

weeks while Actinomycin-D was being given.

4. Actinomycin-D – substituted for Adriamycin after the dose limitation had been reached. The dose of Actinomycin-D was 0.3 mg/m² (top dose limit was 0.5 mg/dose) given on days 1 through 5 of each cycle every 8 weeks. Six courses of Actinomycin-D were given over a period of 1 year. The total time of chemotherapy was 18 months.

Results

Results of this trial were reported when patients had a minimum 9 month followup [16]. Survival rate free of disease at 18 months for patients receiving chemotherapy was 76% compared to 83% for the control group. Extremity and trunk patients were combined in this analysis. In patients with trunk and extremity lesions the overall survival rate at 18 months was 66.7% (18 of 27 patients) for the chemotherapy group and 85% (17 of 20 patients) for the control group. There were two local recurrences in patients in the control group and no local recurrences in patients receiving chemotherapy.

Thus in this study, no evidence was obtained for a positive effect of adjuvant chemotherapy in adult patients with soft tissue sarcomas. A very small number of patients, the short followup, and the combining of patients with diseases at extremity and truncal sites make this a hard study to analyze, however.

Adjuvant Chemotherapy Studies at the National Cancer Institute

Design of the Trials

Since 1975, the Surgery Branch of the National Cancer Institute in conjunction with the Radiation Oncology Branch and the Medical Oncology Branch have been studying the role of adjuvant chemotherapy in the treatment of patients with soft tissue sarcomas of the extremities and head, neck and trunk [5, 17–21]. Between 1975 and 1977, patients with sarcomas were treated in a prospective study with adjuvant chemotherapy consisting of adriamycin, cytoxan, and methotrexate following local therapy with either surgery alone or surgery plus radiation therapy. Because of an apparent improvement in disease free and overall survival in those patients receiving chemotherapy compared to historical controls treated previously at the National Cancer Institute, this historically controlled trial was terminated in June, 1977, and a prospective randomized trial was begun in which patients were randomized to either receive or not receive adjuvant chemotherapy. This prospective randomized trial was terminated in July, 1981, for patients with soft tissue sarcomas of the extremities though the trial is continuing for patients with soft tissue sarcomas of the head, neck and trunk.

In this chapter the results for both the historically controlled trial conducted between May, 1975 and June, 1977 as well as the prospective randomized trial conducted between June, 1977, and July, 1981 will be considered. All patient results are updated as of April 15, 1982. Thus, the minimum followup for patients in the originally historically controlled trial is over four years. The median followup for patients in the prospective randomized trial at the time of analysis was 2-1/2 years. Patients eligible for these protocols had a diagnosis of either round cell or pleomorphic liposarcoma, pleomorphic rhabdomyosarcoma, synovial cell sarcoma, fibrosarcoma, neurofibrosarcoma, leiomyosarcoma, malignant fibrous histiocytoma, or undifferentiated sarcoma. All patients had lesions categorized as grade II or III. Patients eligible for the trials were found to be free of clinical evidence of metastatic disease either in regional lymph nodes or more distant sites following a standard workup including blood chemical analysis, chest x-ray, complete lung tomograms at 1 cm cuts, liver scan, and bone scan. Patients were excluded from the trial if they had received any prior chemotherapy or radiation therapy prior to referral to the National Cancer Institute or if they had a history of any other malignant disease except for basal cell carcinoma. Patients below the age of 30 with a diagnosis of embryonal or alveolar rhabdomyosarcoma were not included in the protocol.

Definitive therapy of local disease was accomplished by either surgery alone or the combination of surgery plus radiation therapy. Patients with extremity lesions received either amputation or limb-sparing wide local resection designed to remove all gross disease. Patients receiving the latter treatment also received radiation therapy to all areas at risk for tumor spread between the joints proximal and distal to the tumor including all involved muscle groups. The radiotherapy techniques involved in the treatment of these patients have been published in detail [22]. In brief, daily treatments at 180 to 200 rads per treatment were given to a total dose of 4500 to 5000 rads. The tumor bed was then treated to a total dose of 6000 to 7000 rads over an additional two week period. An essential feature of treatment was the exclusion of a portion of the circumference of the involved extremity from the treatment portal. Treatment was begun as soon as the wound was healed, generally within two to three weeks following surgery.

The chemotherapy regimen is outlined in Table 2. Patients who received the chemotherapy in conjunction with radiotherapy received the first chemotherapy dose three days prior to the first dose of radiation. The second dose of chemotherapy was given during the radiation therapy treatment and the remaining doses completed after radiation therapy was finished.

All patients in both clinical trials were followed at two monthly intervals with complete physical examination and chest x-rays. Full lung tomography was obtained every six months for three years and yearly thereafter.

Table 2. NCI adjuvant chemotherapy regimen for patients with adult soft tissue sarcomas

Doxorubicin	Day 1 of 28 day treatment cycle, 50 mg/m² i.v. bolus. Escalate each cycle by 10 mg/m² to maximum of 70 mg/m² based on bone marrow tolerance.
Cyclophosphamide	Day 1 of 28 day treatment cycle, 500 mg/m² i.v. drip. Escalate each cycle by 100 mg/m² to maximum of 700 mg/m² based on bone marrow tolerance.

When maximum cumulative doxorubicin dose of 500 to 550 mg/m² is achieved switch to 6 cycles of:

Methotrexate	Day 1 of 28 day treatment cycle, 50 mg/Kg i.v. over 6 hours. Escalate each cycle by 50 mg/Kg to maximum dose of 250 mg/Kg. Citrovorum factor 15 mg/m² i.v. 2 hours after completion of methotrexate and then every 6 hours for 8 doses. Discontinue methotrexate after 6 cycles.

Results of NCI trials for Treatment of Soft Tissue Sarcomas of the Extremities

The results of treatment of 26 consecutive patients with soft tissue sarcomas of the extremities treated between May, 1975 and June, 1977 in a pilot trial in the Surgery Branch of the NCI are shown in Figs. 1 and 2. Minimum followup in this trial is 4–1/2 years. These patients were compared to comparable historical controls at our institution. A marked improvement in protocol patients receiving adjuvant chemotherapy was seen both in the disease-free and overall survival. With all patients followed for 4 years the relapse free 4 year survival rate was 77% in our chemotherapy protocol patients compared to 35% in historical controls. Similarly overall 4-year survivals were 92% in patients treated with chemotherapy and 42% in our historical controls. These differences in both disease-free and overall survival were highly statistically significant (p = .001).

Because of the general unreliability of historically controlled comparisons and our concern, in 1977, that the effects seen in the treatment group might be explained by reasons other than those due to adjuvant chemotherapy, a prospective randomized trial was initiated in which patients were randomized to either receive or not receive this chemotherapy. Between June, 1977 and July, 1981, 65 patients with soft tissue sarcomas of the extremities were randomized into this treatment protocol. Details of the site, histology, grade, age, type of surgery and final resection margin for these patients are presented in Table 3. A dramatic improvement was seen in patients randomized to receive adjuvant chemotherapy (Table 4, and Figs. 3 and 4). There were three recurrences and one death in 37 patients randomized to receive chemotherapy and 9 recurrences and

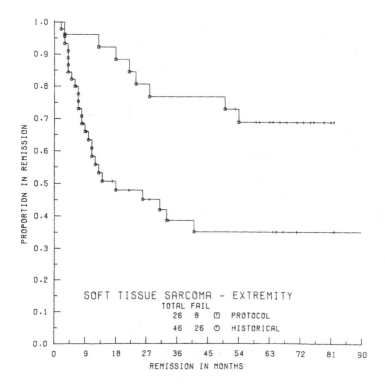

Fig. 1. Trial of adjuvant chemotherapy for adult patients with soft tissue sarcomas of the extremities conducted in Surgery Branch of the NCI between 1975 and 1977. Minimum followup in the trial is 4–1/2 years. Substantial improvement was seen in disease-free remission in patients receiving adjuvant chemotherapy compared to historical controls (p = .001).

4 deaths in 28 patients randomized to receive no chemotherapy. An advantage in both continuous disease-free survival (p = .0008) and in overall survival (p = .04) was seen in patients randomized to receive chemotherapy. Three year actuarial disease-free survival for patients randomized to receive chemotherapy was 92% compared to 60% for patients randomized to receive no chemotherapy. The actuarial three year overall survival for patients receiving chemotherapy was 95% compared to 74% for patients receiving no chemotherapy. These results strongly indicate that adjuvant chemotherapy with this regimen was of benefit to patients with soft tissue sarcomas of the extremities. Further followup is, of course, necessary and this is continuing. On the basis of this trial, however, it is recommended that all patients with extremity soft tissue sarcomas receive adjuvant chemotherapy with a regimen containing doxorubicin.

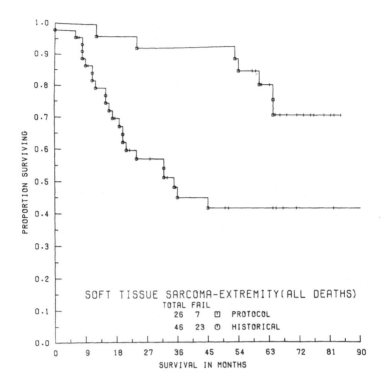

Fig. 2. Trial of adjuvant chemotherapy for adult patients with soft tissue sarcomas of the extremities conduced in the Surgery Branch of the NCI between 1975 and 1977. Minimum followup in the trial is 4–1 = 2 years. Substantial improvement was seen in overall survival in patients receiving adjuvant chemotherapy compared to historical controls (p = .001).

Results of NCI Trials for Treatment of Soft Tissue Sarcomas of the Head, Neck and Trunk

Our studies of adjuvant chemotherapy in patients with head, neck and truncal lesions, however, have indicated no benefit of adjuvant chemotherapy either in our retrospective historically controlled trial or in our prospective randomized trial. Of the 24 patients randomized to receive chemotherapy there were 9 failures and 7 deaths. Of the 16 patients randomized to receive no chemotherapy there were 4 recurrences and 3 deaths (p_2 = .33 and .22, respectively). The wide diversity of anatomic locations in the head, neck, retroperitoneum, mediastinum and abdominal wall make this group quite heterogeneous. There are not enough patients in any specific anatomic site to determine whether or not adjuvant chemotherapy is of benefit in any subgroup of these patients. The difference between the effectiveness of adjuvant chemotherapy in patients with extremity

Table 3. Soft tissue sarcomas of the extremity (Number of patients in percentage).

		Chemotherapy	No chemotherapy	Total
Total		37	28	65
Site	Arm	5 (13)	5 (18)	10 (15)
	Forearm and hand	7 (19)	3 (11)	10 (15)
	Thigh	17 (46)	16 (57)	33 (51)
	Leg and foot	8 (22)	4 (14)	12 (19)
Histology	Fibrosarcoma	0 (0)	4 (15)	5 (8)
	Malignant fibrous histiocytoma	9 (24)	9 (33)	18 (27)
	Liposarcoma	5 (14)	6 (21)	11 (17)
	Leiomyosarcoma	2 (5)	2 (7)	4 (6)
	Rhabdomyosarcoma	2 (5)	0 (0)	2 (3)
	Synovial sarcoma	12 (33)	4 (14)	16 (24)
	Neurofibrosarcoma	3 (8)	2 (7)	5 (8)
	Unclassified	4 (11)	1 (3)	5 (7)
Grade	1	0 (0)	0 (0)	0 (0)
	2	6 (16)	8 (29)	14 (22)
	3	31 (84)	20 (71)	51 (78)
Age	0–20	4 (11)	5 (18)	9 (14)
	21–40	17 (46)	10 (36)	27 (41)
	41–60	15 (41)	9 (32)	24 (36)
	>60	1 (2)	4 (14)	5 (8)
Surgery	Amputation	16 (43)	11 (39)	27 (42)
	Limb-sparing	21 (57)	17 (61)	38 (58)
Final resection margin	Negative	33 (89)	26 (93)	59 (90)
	Positive	3 (8)	0 (0)	3 (5)
	Unknown	1 (3)	2 (7)	3 (5)

lesions and in patients with head, neck and trunk lesions can probably be attributed to the different patterns of local spread for lesions in these two locations. It is extremely difficult to provide effective local control for many patients with head, neck and truncal lesions and the amount of microscopic residual disease following surgical resection is probably larger in these patients then in patients with extremity sarcomas.

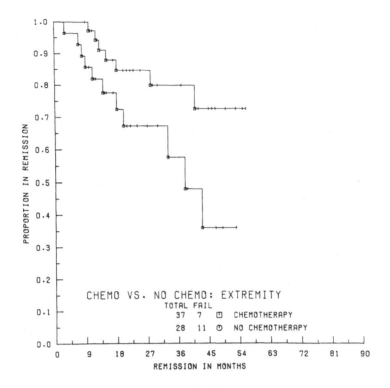

Fig. 3. A prospective randomized trial comparing the use of chemotherapy to that of no chemothera-py in adult patients with soft tissue sarcomas of the extremities. Patients randomized to receive chemotherapy had a significantly improved continuous disease-free survival (p = .0008).

Other Studies of Adjuvant Chemotherapy in Patients with Soft Tissue Sarcomas

A prospective randomized study of adjuvant chemotherapy in adult patients with soft tissue sarcomas is being performed at the Mayo Clinic in Rochester, Minnesota though results have been reported in abstract form only [23]. In this trial patients are being randomized to receive either chemotherapy or no chemo-therapy. The chemotherapy consists of vincristine, cyclophosphamide and dacti-nomycin alternated at 6 week intervals with vincristine, doxorubicin and dacar-bazine. Preliminary reports indicated that hematogeneous metastases were less frequent in patients randomized to receive chemotherapy [23]. Hematogeneous metastases were seen in one of 30 patients receiving adjuvant chemotherapy compared to 7 of 31 patients not receiving chemotherapy (p < .05). However, no significant treatment related differences in overall recurrence or survival rates had been seen at the time of this preliminary report.

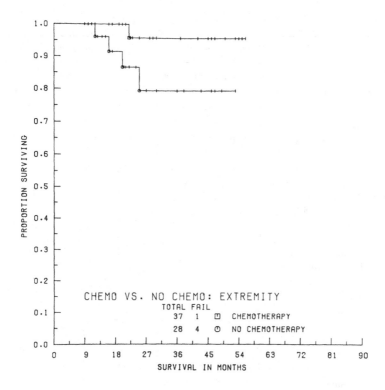

Fig. 4. A prospective randomized trial comparing the use of chemotherapy to that of no chemotherapy in adult patients with soft tissue sarcomas of the extremities. Patients randomized to receive chemotherapy had a significantly improved overall survival (p = .04).

Recently, several reports of noncontrolled trials utilizing adjuvant chemotherapy for adult patients with soft tissue sarcomas have suggested that adjuvant chemotherapy may be effective in reducing recurrence and prolonging survival. These reports represent historically controlled trials and conclusions from them must therefore be taken with some caution. Sordillo *et al.* at Memorial Sloan Kettering Hospital reported on the treatment of 64 adult patients with soft tissue sarcomas receiving adjuvant chemotherapy with a 6 drug regimen [24]. The chemotherapy regimen used is seen in Table 5.

With a median followup of 50 months, 19 patients relapsed, 9 with local recurrence at the surgical site and 10 with metastatic tumor in the lungs. These results were somewhat better than would be expected on the basis of historical controls. In addition, a 58% recurrence rate was seen in 12 patients who discontinued therapy early because of nausea compared to the 23% recurrence rate of patients who completed or relapsed on therapy. This significant difference

Table 4. Soft tissue sarcomas of the extremities (Number of patients in percentage).

		Chemotherapy			No chemotherapy		
		n	Recurred	Dead	n	Recurred	Dead
Total		37	7	1	28	11	4
Site	Arm	5	1	0	5	1	0
	Forearm and hand	7	0	0	3	2	0
	Thigh	17	5	1	16	7	3
	Leg and foot	8	1	0	4	1	1
Histology	Fibrosarcoma	0	3	0	4	3	1
	Malignant fibrous histiocytoma	9	1	1	9	1	0
	Liposarcoma	5	0	0	6	2	1
	Leiomyosarcoma	2	1	0	2	1	1
	Rhabdomyosarcoma	2	0	0	0	0	0
	Synocial sarcoma	12	1	0	4	3	1
	Neurofibrosarcoma	3	0	0	2	0	0
	Unclassified	4	1	0	1	1	0
Grade	1	0	0	0	0	0	0
	2	6	1	0	8	2	1
	3	31	6	1	20	9	3
Surgery	Amputation	16	5	1	11	6	2
	Limb-sparing	21	2	0	27	5	2

Table 5. ALOMAD chemotherapy regimen for soft tissue sarcomas

The chemotherapy schedule consisted of six 84-day cycles at the following dosages:

Day 1	Vincristine 1.0 mg/m^2 iv, followed in 1 to 4 h by methotrexate 250 mg/m^2 i.v. over 2 h.
Day 2	Citrovorum factor 50 mg/m^2, adriamycin 40 mg/m^2 and dacarbazine 500 mg/m^2, all given i.v. push, followed in 4 to 8 h by citrovorum 5 mg po. q 8 h × 6 doses.
Day 15	Start leukeran 6 mg/m^2/day, po × 14 days.
Day 22	Actinomycin D 1.2 mg/m^2 i.v. push.
Day 29	Discontinue leukeran.
Day 43	Adriamycin 50 mg/m^2 i.v. push.
Day 57	Resume leukeran 6 mg/m^2/day po × 14 days.
Day 64	Actinomycin D 1.2 mg/m^2 i.v. push.
Day 71	Discontinue leukeran.
Day 85	Recycle.

From Sordillo *et al.* [5]

(p = .01) led these workers to believe that the differences seen in patients treated with chemotherapy were real and not due to differences in patient selection.

Das Gupta *et al.* at the University of Illinois Medical Center treated 113 adult patients with soft tissue sarcomas with adjuvant chemotherapy consisting of adriamycin, 60 mg/m² intravenously on day 1 and DTIC, 250 mg/m² on days 1 through 5 repeated every 22 days to a total adriamycin dose of 500 mg/m² [25]. Seventy-seven percent of patients receiving adjuvant chemotherapy lived disease-free for 2 years compared to a concurrent, but nonrandomized group of 144 patients with a disease-free survival at 2 years at 59%. Of the patients eligible for five-year survival analysis in the chemotherapy group 74% were disease-free compared to 50% in the group treated by surgery alone. These results suggested that adjuvant chemotherapy was of benefit though the diversity of patients with soft tissue sarcomas and the possible selection criteria involved in treating patients by one strategy or another could account for these differences.

Several groups have reported the use of intrarterial adriamycin [26–31] prior to limb-sparing surgery in patients with soft tissue sarcomas with an apparent improvement in continuous disease-free and overall survival in patients treated by this modality compared to historical controls treated without chemotherapy. Further work is necessary to determine whether intra-arterial administration of adriamycin is superior to the administration of this drug by the more conventional intravenous approach.

Summary

The rarity and heterogeneity of adult soft tissue sarcomas in adults has made it difficult to perform critical studies of the role of adjuvant chemotherapy in these patients. It appears, on the basis of recent evidence, that adjuvant chemotherapy is of benefit in prolonging disease-free and overall survival in patients with soft tissue sarcomas of the extremities and this treatment is recommended for patients with extremity lesions. it has not been possible to demonstrate a benefit of adjuvant chemotherapy in patients with soft tissue sarcomas of the head, neck and trunk.

References

1. Patten BM: Human Embryology. New York: McGraw-Hill, 1968.
2. Hajdu SI: Pathology of Soft Tissue Tumors. Philadelphia: Lea and Feiger, 1979.
3. Enzinger FM: Recent developments in the classification of soft tissue sarcomas. In: Management of Primary Bone and Soft Tissue Tumors. Chicago: Year Book Medical Publishers, 1977.
4. Russell WO, Cohen J, Enzinger FM *et al.*: A clinical and pathological staging system for soft tissue sarcomas. Cancer 40:1562–1570, 1977.

5. Rosenberg SA, Kent H, Costa J et al.: Prospective randomized evaluation of the role of limb-sparing surgery, radiation therapy, and adjuvant chemoimmunotherapy in the treatment of adult soft-tissue sarcomas. Surgery 84:62–69, 1978.

6. Gerner RE, Moore GE, Pickren JW: Soft tissue sarcomas. Ann Surg 181:803–808, 1975.

7. Shieber W, Graham P: An experience with sarcomas of the soft tissues in adults. Surgery 52:295, 1962.

8. Martin RG, Butler JJ, Albores-Saavedra J: Soft tissue tumors: Surgical treatment and results. In: Tumors of Bone and Soft Tissue. Chicago: Year Book Medical Publishers, 1965.

9. Pack GI, Ariel IM: Treatment of cancer and allied diseases. In: Tumors of the Soft Somatic Tissues and Bone, Vol. VIII. New York: Harper and Row, 1964.

10. Hare HF, Cerny MF: Soft tissue sarcoma: A review of 200 cases. Cancer 16:1332, 1963.

11. Shiu MH, Castro EB, Hajdu SI et al.: Surgical treatment of 297 soft tissue sarcomas of the lower extremity. Ann Surg 182:597, 1975.

12. Cantin J, McNeer GP, Chu FC et al.: The problem of local recurrence after treatment of soft tissue sarcoma. Ann Surg 168:47–53, 1968.

13. Simon MA, Enneking WF: The management of soft-tissue sarcomas of the extremities. J Bone Joint Surg 58-A:317, 1976.

14. Lindberg RD, Martin RG, Romsdahl MM: Surgery and postoperative radiotherapy in the treatment of soft tissue sarcomas in adults. Am J Roentgenol Rad Therap Nucl Med 123:123–129, 1975.

15. Chang AE, Schaner EG, Conkle DM et al.: Evaluation of computed tomography in the detection of pulmonary metastases: A prospective study. Cancer 43:913–916, 1979.

16. Lindberg RD, Murphy WK, Benjamin RS et al.: Adjuvant chemotherapy in the treatment of soft tissue sarcomas: A preliminary study. In: M.D. Anderson Hospital and Tumor Institute (ed), Management of Primary Bone and Soft Tissue Tumors. Chicago: Year Book Medical Publishers, 1977.

17. Rosenberg SA, Glatstein EJ: Perspectives on the role of surgery and radiation therapy in the treatment of soft tissue sarcomas of the extremities. Semin Oncol 8:190–200, 1981.

18. Rosenberg SA, Tepper J, Glatstein E et al.: Adjuvant chemotherapy for patients with soft tissue sarcomas. Surg Clin North Am 61:1415–1423, 1981.

19. Sugarbaker PH, Barofsky I, Rosenberg SA et al.: Quality of life assessment of patients in extremity sarcoma clinical trials. Surgery 91:17–23, 1982.

20. Rosenberg SA, Tepper J, Glatstein E: Prospective randomized evaluation of adjuvant chemotherapy in adults with soft tissue sarcomas of the extremities. Cancer, in press.

21. Dresdale A, Bonow RO, Wesley R et al.: Prospective evaluation of doxorubicin-induced cardiomyopathy resulting from post-surgical adjuvant treatment of patients with soft tissue sarcomas. Cancer, in press.

22. Tepper J, Glatstein E, Rosenberg SA: Radiation therapy technique in soft tissue sarcomas of the extremity. Intl J Radiat Oncol Biol Phys, in press.

23. Edmonson JH, Fleming TR, Ivins JC et al.: Reduced hematogenous metastasis in patients who receive systemic chemotherapy following excision of soft tissue sarcomas: Preliminary report. Clin Invest 193, 1980.

24. Sordillo PP, Magill GB, Shiu MH et al.: Adjuvant chemotherapy of soft-part sarcomas with ALOMAD (S4). J Surg Oncol 18:345–353, 1981.

25. Das Gupta TK, Patel MK, Chaudhuri PK et al.: The role of chemotherapy as an adjuvant to surgery in the initial treatment of primary soft tissue sarcomas in adults. J Surg Oncol 19:139–144, 1982.

26. Yonemoto RH, Byron RL, Jacobs ML: Combined irradiation, intra-arterial chemotherapy, and surgery for the treatment of sarcomas of the extremities. Surgery 61:355–360, 1967.

27. Haskell CM, Silverstein MJ, Rangel DM et al.: Multimodality cancer therapy in man: A pilot

study of adriamycin by arterial infusion. Cancer 33:1485–1490, 1972.

28. Didolkar MS, Kanter PM, Baffi RR *et al.*: Comparison of regional versus systemic chemotherapy with adriamycin. Ann Surg 187:332–336, 1978.

29. Karakousis CP, Lopez R, Catane R *et al.*: Intraarterial adriamycin in the treatment of soft tissue sarcomas. J Surg Oncol 13:21–27, 1980.

30. Weisenburger TH, Eilber FR, Grant TT *et al.*: Multidisciplinary 'limb salvage' treatment of soft tissue and skeletal sarcomas. Int J Radiat Oncol Biol Phys 7:1495–1499, 1981.

31. Lokich JJ: Preoperative chemotherapy in soft tissue sarcoma. Surg Gynecol Obstet 148:512–516, 1979.

7. Perfusion Chemotherapy*

FREDERICK R. EILBER

The treatment of adult soft tissue sarcomas remains an extremely confusing and difficult problem. These tumors often present as very large lesions with very few local or systemic symptoms and often are misdiagnosed and treated as 'chronic hematomas' or muscle group ruptures for a long period of time. Furthermore, there is confusion in pathologic nomenclature of these tumors and the biologic importance of the various histogenic varieties. The original work by Lattes and Stout, which separated these tumors into the cell of origin, was a major step toward their systemic categorization [1, 2]; however, because these tumors are often undifferentiated, it has been very difficult for pathologists to reach agreement on the histogenic cell of origin, i.e., a rhabdomyosarcoma versus synovial cell sarcoma. Recently, the American Joint Committee on Staging and End Results proposed a clinical pathological grading system that appeared to accurately predict overal survival in a retrospective review [3]. In this system the grade of tumor was established by determining the number of mitoses per high-power field; a high-grade tumor would display the greatest number of mitoses. Retrospectively, they could show that patients with Grade III tumors treated by surgery alone had less than a 20% 5-year survival rate.

The local biology of these tumors also presents many difficult problems. In addition to the large mass effect, these tumors can extend along fascial planes for long distances, often with normal intervening tissues. This extension capability poses problems in terms of radiation therapy or surgical excision of all gross tumor. Although these tumors do compress vessels or nerves and become intimately associated with bone, they rarely directly invade these structures. The final difficulty has to do with delineating which types of tumors have the greatest metastatic potential and, therefore, pose the greatest threat to the patient. These tumors appear to spread through the bloodstream to the chest and, rarely, to lymph nodes. An exception to this route would be the retroperitoneal sarcomas, which have a high metastatic potential to the liver.

At the present time, three major factors are related to overal prognosis: (1)

* Supported by grants CA29605 and CB04344, awarded by the National Cancer Institute, DHEW.

Baker, L.H. (ed.), Soft Tissue Sarcomas. ISBN 0-89838-584-9

local control of the tumor, (2) size of the original lesion, and (3) grade of the tumor.

History of Prior Therapy

Surgical excision is the treatment of choice for patients with soft tissue sarcomas. However, experience with various types of surgical procedures has shown that local excision results in local failure approximately 95% of the time [4], and that extended operations such as muscle group excision or compartment excision improved the local control to approximately 40% [5]. Finally, in a series that involves amputations, the local recurrence rate was further reduced to approximately 35% [6]. The probable reason for the continued high local failure rate, even with major amputation, again has to do with the biology of the tumor. Because these tumors often are large and proximally placed in the thigh or arm, a wide excision margin is difficult even with major amputation.

In 1968, several investigators began to study the effects of radiation therapy for adult soft tissue sarcomas. Early experience with orthovoltage or megavoltage radiation produced very little response in the gross tumor masses [7]. Thus these tumors earned a reputation for being 'radio-resistant.' However, both Suit *et al.* and Lindberg *et al.* concluded that if only microscopic residual disease could be treated, a greater therapeutic index might be obtained [8, 9, 10]. Their conclusion was borne out by sequential studies of patients who received between 5,000 and 6,000 rads of radiation therapy following a local excision of their tumor. Several studies from M.D. Anderson and, more recently, from Massachusetts General Hospital report that local control of these tumors can be obtained in approximately 85% of the patients without amputation [11]. This improved local control rate could be translated into improved overall survival of patients in these series compared to historical groups treated with primary surgical procedures. Despite the fact that radiation therapy creates some significant long-term problems such as fibrosis and joint stiffness, if does appear to be a feasible method for preservation of a functional extremity [12].

With the advent of chemotherapy, several investigators began to study the effects of infusion or perfusion of these cytotoxic agents into soft tissue sarcomas. The concept of regional intraarterial chemotherapy was suggested by Clopp in 1950, and the technique of isolation perfusion of an extremity was introduced first by Creech in 1957 and altered to hyperthermic isolated limb perfusion in 1967 by Stehlin [13, 14]. The basic premise of this therapy was to deliver high concentrations of drug into an extremity that had been excluded from the systemic circulation by a tourniquet technique. In this way, a higher cytotoxic concentration could be delivered to the tumor and to the extremity without risk to the remainder of the body or, more specifically, the bone marrow.

These trials used L-Pam and Actinomycin-D. In 1975, Stehlin reported results with 37 patients treated with isolation limb perfusion from 1957 to 1975 [15]. Seventeen of the 37 also received 3000 rads of radiation therapy to the tumor bed preoperatively before their limb perfusion with L-Pam and Actinomycin-D for 2.5 hours at temperature up to 43°. Of these 37 patients, two died, two had amputations, and six had local recurrence (17%) with an overall 61% survival. McBride and Krementz also reported similar results for isolated limb perfusion [16, 17].

This limb perfusion technique is extremely interesting and presents some theoretical advantages for delivery of high concentration of drug to a tumor; however, it also presents some major logistic and practical problems. The technique is limited, necessarily, to patients with extremity tumors in the distal two-thirds of the thigh or arm because of the tourniquet replacement. Thus, the patient with a proximal thigh or arm tumor, or patients with retroperitoneal sarcomas or head and neck lesions, must receive another type of treatment. From a practicality standpoint, this technique requires a long time in the operating room and at least 2.5 hours on a cardio-pulmonary pump oxygenator in order to maintain a viable extremity.

The technique and the reports did, however, stimulate several investigators to consider using preoperative therapy.

The concept of presurgical treatment of sarcomas is an attractive one. Clearly, there are two major problems for local control – the periphery of the tumor and the microscopic extensions beyond the gross tumor mass. Treatment with chemotherapy before the blood supply is interrupted and/or treatment with radiation, especially the peripheral cells when they are in a relatively oxic state, would seem to offer many theoretic advantages. The most effective preoperative chemotherapeutic agent for the adult soft tissue sarcoma is Adriamycin [18]. Unfortunately, it is not possible to use this drug for isolated limb perfusion because it induces marked tissue necrosis even with reduced dosages.

Multidisciplinary Preoperative Therapy

With the above background, we began a series of pilot studies to determine if it was possible to obtain histologic evidence of tumor cell destruction by preoperative therapy. We reasoned that if we could induce necrosis, then we could perform localized operative procedures and improve local disease control. In the original pilot study, we used intraarterial Adriamycin given not by the isolated limb perfusion technique but by an infusion [19]. Percutaneous intraarterial catheters were placed by the Seldinger technique into the major arterial supply to the tumor. Adriamycin was infused at a rate of 30 mg/day over 24 h for 3 consecutive days. In an original series of 10 patients, this technique was shown to be not only logistically feasible, but no serious vascular complications ensued. With the original four patients we found that Heparin could not be added to the perfusate because the Adriamycin precipitated. Our second lesson came when we found that the catheter tip needed to be placed in a high flow vessel, such as the common femoral artery or axillary artery, because placement in smaller caliber vessels close to the size of the indwelling line, such as the brachial or popliteal, caused marked skin erythema and muscle necrosis. Finally, we found that an injection of fluorescein and the use of a Woods Lamp allowed us to assess the distribution of flow through the arterial line.

When these preoperatively treated tumors were examined after resection, approximately 50% of the tumor cells showed necrosis. This judgment was made by a single pathologist who assessed the absence of nuclei in cells per high power field based on a grid technique.

We based these pilot studies on the fact that radiation was most effective for microscopic disease and that the Adriamycin was a very effective radiation sensitizer. We reasoned that by adding radiation immediately after the infusion of Adriamycin, an additional cytotoxic effect could be obtained. Furthermore, there was some experimental evidence suggesting that higher dose fractions of 350 rads/day vs. 200 rads/day might be more effective for soft tissue sarcomas because of the 'shoulder effect' seen with some of these tumors in culture.

Therefore, the next 10 patients were treated with intraarterial Adriamycin at the same dose, and immediately following removal of the intraarterial line received 350 rads/day for 10 treatment days over a 2-week period [20, 21]. It must be mentioned that the entire extremity was treated to encompass the muscle groups from their origin to insertion. A strip of skin was spared opposite the primary tumor and/or biopsy site. Approximately 1 week later, or 3 weeks following the initiation of therapy, these patients received radical en bloc (but still local) resection of their tumor mass. In this series of patients, we found that the tumor cell necrosis had increased to approximately 85% in the resected specimens. There were few intraoperative problems and very little radiation fibrosis or tissue reaction as a result of preoperative therapy. However, in the original series of 10 patients treated with this regimen, two patients had marked wound necrosis from attempts to close the primary wound by placing irradiated skin under tension. We also found that clinically there were no objective responses, or a 50% reduction in tumor size, in 90% of these patients.

Since 1975, a third consecutive series of 107 patients has been treated with preoperative intraarterial Adriamycin and radiation therapy followed by radical en bloc excision of tumor [21, 22]. To date, three patients (2.5%) have had evidence of a local recurrence with an overall survival rate of 65%. It must be mentioned that all patients had lesions greater than 5 cm in diameter with 60% having lesions greater than 10 cm, and all lesions were pathologic Grade III. Of these patients, two required amputation because of complications of therapy, but the overall limb salvage rate was greater than 98%.

Recently, there have been other reports of infusions using additional chemotherapeutic agents. Karakousis from Roswell Park has infused Adriamycin – 10–20 mg – and Methotrexate – 10 mg per intraarterial line – with no major complications using a pneumatic tourniquet [23].

Chuang and Benjamin used intraarterial cis-Platinum in 10 patients with malignant sarcomas of bone at dosages of 120 mg/m^2 over a 2-hour period every 3–4 weeks [24]. They reported that 5/7 patients had either partial or complete remission of their disease. Although these studies are early pilot trials, they show considerable promise. Continued investigations of the intraarterial route to obtain higher concentrations and/or an improved therapeutic index for chemotherapeutic agents is justified as an area of active research.

Summary

The major factors influencing prognosis for patients with adult soft tissue sarcoma are local disease control, size of the primary tumor, and the grade of the primary lesion. Since grade and tumor size are variables that are difficult, if not impossible, to control in a clinical setting, additional efforts must be concentrated to improve local disease control. Preoperative therapy consisting of regional chemotherapy and radiation therapy has been shown to be a highly effective method for improving local disease control. Obviously, this multidisciplinary therapy is not necessary for all patients with adult soft tissue sarcomas because those with small, well differentiated tumors can be adequately treated by surgery alone. However, those patients with large, high grade tumors or tumors located in the head and neck or retroperitoneum. where surgical excision is much more difficult, would benefit from a multidisciplinary preoperative therapy. The local disease control rate of over 98% in a consecutive series of 110 patients with extremity soft tissue sarcomas treated by intraarterial Adriamycin, radiation therapy, and surgical excision attests to the effectiveness of this therapy. In order to make the treatment more universally effective and applicable, several studies are being conducted to determine whether it is absolutely essential to use the intraarterial route rather than an intravenous route for Adriamycin and whether the dose rate fraction is the proper one.

Clearly, the next 10 years should see some exciting therapeutic changes for patients with adult soft tissue sarcomas, not only in the preservation of a functional extremity but, more importantly, in the achievement of local disease control, which will affect the overall survival rate.

106

References

1. Stout AP: Sarcomas of the soft tissue. Cancer 11:210, 1961.
2. Stout AP, Lattes R: Tumors of the soft tissue. In: Atlas of Tumor Pathology, 2nd Series, Fasicle I, Washington, AFIP, 1967.
3. Russell WO, Cohen J, Enzinger F, *et al.*: A clinical and pathological staging system for soft tissue sarcoma. Cancer 40:1562–1570, 1977.
4. Bowden L, Booher RJ: The principles and techniques of resection of soft parts for sarcoma. Surgery 44:963, 1958.
5. Shiu MH, Castrol EB, Hajdu SI, Fortner JG: Surgical treatment of 297 soft tissue sarcomas of the lower extremity, Ann Surg 182:597–602, 1975.
6. Martin RG, Butler JJ, Albores-Saavedra J: Soft tissue tumors: Surgical treatment and results. In: Tumor of Bone and Soft Tissue, Chicago, Year Book Medical Publishers, 1965, pp 333–347.
7. Gilbert HA, Kagan RA, Winkley J: Soft tissue sarcomas of the extremities: Their natural history, treatment and radiation sensitivity. J Surg Oncol 7:303–317, 1975.
8. Suit HD, Russell WO, Martin RG: Management of patients with sarcoma of soft tissue in an extremity. Cancer 31:1247–1255, 1973.
9. Suit HD, Russell WO, Martin RG: Sarcoma of soft tissue: Clinical and histopathological parameters and response to treatment. Cancer 35:1478–1483, 1975.
10. Lindberg RD, Murphy WK: Adjuvant chemotherapy in the treatment of primary soft tissue sarcomas. In: Management of Primary Bone and Soft Tissue Tumors. Chicago: Year Book Medical Publications, 1977, pp 343–352.
11. Suit HD, Proppe KH, Mankin HJ, Wood WC: Preoperative radiation therapy for sarcoma of soft tissue. Cancer 47:2269–2274, 1981.
12. Rosenberg SA, Kent H, Costa J, *et al.*: Prospective randomized evaluation of the role of limb sparing surgery, radiation, and adjuvant chemotherapy in the treatment of adult soft tissue sarcomas. Surgery 84:62–69, 1978.
13. Stehlin J Jr: Hyperthermic perfusion with chemotherapy for cancers of the extremities. Surg Gynecol Obstet 129:305–308, 1969.
14. Stehlin JS Jr: Regional chemotherapy for soft tissue sarcomas. In: Tumors of Bone and Soft Tissue. Chicago: Year Book Medical Publishers, 1965, pp 367–374.
15. Stehlin JS, de Ipoli PD, Giovanella BC, Guiterrez AE, Anderson RF: Soft tissue sarcomas of the extremity: Multidisciplinary therapy employing hyperthermic perfusion. Am J Surg 130:643–646, 1975.
16. McBride CM: Sarcoma of the limb: Results of adjuvant chemotherapy using isolated limb perfusion. Arch Surg 109:304–308, 1974.
17. McBride CM: Regional chemotherapy for soft tissue sarcomas. In: Management of Primary Bone and Soft Tissue Tumors. Chicago: Year Book Medical Publishers, 1977, pp 353–360.
18. Tan C, Etcubanas E, Wollner N, Rosen G, Gilladoga A, Showell J, Murphy ML, Knakoff IH: Adriamycin – an antitumor antibiotic in the treatment of neoplastic disease. Cancer 32:9–17, 1973.
19. Haskell CM, Eilber FR, Morton DL: Adriamycin (NSC-123127) by arterial infusion. Cancer Chemother Rep 6:187–189, 1975.
20. Morton DL, Eilber FR, Townsend CM Jr, Grant TT, Mirra J, Weisenburger TH: Limb salvage from a multidisciplinary treatment approach for skeletal and soft tissue sarcomas of the extremity. Ann Surg 184:268–278, 1976.
21. Eilber FR, Townsend CM, Weisenburger TH, Mirra JM, Morton DL: Preoperative intraarterial adriamycin and radiation therapy for extremity soft tissue sarcomas: A clinicopathologic study. In: Management of Primary Bone and Soft Tissue Tumors. Chicago: Year Book Medical Publishers, 1977, pp 411–422.

22. Eilber FR, Mirra J, Grant TT, Weisenberger TH, Morton DL: Is amputation necessary for extremity sarcomas? A seven-year experience with limb salvage. Ann Surg 192:431–437, 1980.
23. Karakousis CP, Rao U, Holtermann OA, Kanter PM, Holyoke ED: Tourniquet infusion chemotherapy in extremities with malignant lesions. Surg Gynecol Obstet 481–490, 1979.
24. Chuang VP, Wallace S, Benjamin RS, Jaffee N: Therapeutic intraarterial infusion of cis-Platinum in the management of malignant bone tumors. A preliminary report. Invest Radiol 14:364, 1979.

8. Infusion Chemotherapy for Soft Tissue Sarcomas

ROBERT S. BENJAMIN and BOH-SENG YAP

Introduction

Adriamycin has formed the backbone of sarcoma chemotherapy since its in-troduction into clinical practice. The pioneering studies in this field by the late Dr. Jeffrey Gottlieb demonstrated modest but definite improvement in response rate, remission duration and survival when Adriamycin was combined with DIC and slight further improvement with the addition of cyclophosphamide [1–5]. Other drugs have been relatively ineffective, and the CyVADIC regimen, in-troduced in 1973, remains the standard of sarcoma chemotherapy [3–5]. Review of the data from our own institution from 1973–1977 revealed an 18% complete remission rate and a 49% complete plus partial remission rate in 169 patients treated with the CyVADIC regimen [6]. Patients who achieve complete remis-sion have the potential for long term survival, and this is true whether the complete remission is a response to chemotherapy alone or to chemotherapy and surgery [7]. Unfortunately, maintenance chemotherapy without adriamycin has been ineffective, and the majority of patients relapse after adriamycin has been discontinued to prevent cardiac toxicity.

Since adriamycin is central to the management of patients with sarcomas, we reasoned that we might be able to prolong remission duration and survival by prolonging the duration of adriamycin therapy. Using a standard schedule of adriamycin administration, cardiotoxic doses are usually reached after 6–9 courses of chemotherapy. We therefore proposed to explore the effects of 12–18 courses of chemotherapy utilizing a less cardiotoxic, continuous-infusion regi-men. Our studies on the cardiotoxicity of continuous-infusion adriamycin have demonstrated that substantially higher adriamycin doses may be given by the continuous-infusion schedule than by the standard, intermittent, single-dose, rapid-infusion schedule [8]. Not only can the dose of adriamycin be almost doubled, but the resulting cardiac damage as assessed by endomyocardial biopsy is still less.

We therefore designed a study with two objectives: to increase complete re-misson rate by planned surgical resection of residual disease after three courses

Baker, L.H. (ed.), Soft Tissue Sarcomas. ISBN 0-89838-584-9

© 1983 Martinus Nijhoff Publishers, Boston/The Hague/Dordrecht/Lancaster. Printed in the Netherlands.

of chemotherapy, and to increase remission duration by continuing adriamycin for up to 18 months by using the continuous-infusion schedule. Since our previous studies have demonstrated that vincristine did not add substantially to the CyVADIC regimen, we utilized only CyADIC. Cyclophosphamide was given as an initial infusion on day 1 at a dose of 600 mg/m², usually infused over 4 h in one liter of normal saline. Thereafter, adriamycin and DIC were mixed together and infused daily over 24 h for 4 days in total doses of 60 mg/m² for the adriamycin and 1000 mg/m² for DIC. Prior to institution of this study, we determined the compatability and stability of the two drugs together. To prevent extravasation, all drugs were delivered through indwelling silastic central venous catheters placed percutaneously from the antecubital fossa or the subclavian vein. The catheters were left in place as long as the patient continued on chemotherapy for up to two years. Rarely, they required removal due to infection and/or due to technical complications. Usually, a new catheter could be reinserted into the same vein by first placing a guidewire through the original catheter before its withdrawal. Constant infusion was insured utilizing a continuous infusion pump. Most infusions were performed on an outpatient basis using the Autosyringe AS2F portable pump. Hospital infusions were managed using the Imed pump.

Treatment was initiated at the first level as noted above; however, doses of adriamycin and cyclophosphamide were increased regardless of myelosuppression unless there was infection or moderately severe mucositis (Table 1). Sixty percent of patients tolerated treatment well at the first level and had their doses escalated to the second level. Twenty-five percent had doses increased to the third level. In two-thirds of these cases, however, dosage reduction to the second level was necessary because of severe mucositis. Treatment was usually repeated at 4-week intervals. If cumulative myelosuppression or thrombocytopenia was observed, the dose of DIC was selectively reduced. If significant neutropenia and infection was encountered at the first level, cyclophosphamide was deleted and DIC reduced so that the dose of adriamycin could be maintained at 60 mg/m² in almost all cases.

Fifty patients with soft tissue sarcomas have been entered on the study and followed for at least one year. The group was evenly divided between males and females, and the median age was 42 with a range of 16–75. Fifty-two percent of the patients had distant metastases, usually in lung. The remainder had advanced, local disease. Histologic material was reviewed at our institution in all cases. The most frequent diagnosis was malignant fibrous histiocytoma occurring in 26% of patients. Neurogenic sarcomas occurred in 12% of patients, and angiosarcoma, leiomyosarcoma and unclassified sarcoma each occurred in 10% of patients.

Table 1. Continuous infusion CyADIC.

Drug	Schedule	Total dose/Course in mg/m^2		
		Dose levels		
		1	2	3
Cyclophosphamide	Day 1	600	750	900
Adriamycin	4-Day infusion	60	75	90
Dacarbazine (DIC)	4-Day infusion	1000	1000	1000

Results

The response to chemotherapy on the continuous-infusion program was evaluated after three courses of chemotherapy to determine whether the patient was a candidate for surgical resection of all disease to achieve complete remission. Those who were not surgical condidates continued on chemotherapy or were taken off study depending upon response. Of the 50 patients, 7 or 14% achieved complete remission through chemotherapy alone (Table 2). Twenty patients achieved partial remission for an overall complete plus partial remission rate of 54%. Four patients showed improvement or minor response, 9 had stable disease and ten or 20% progressed in spite of chemotherapy. Complete remissions were seen in patients with malignant fibrous histiocytoma, neurogenic sarcoma, angiosarcoma, rhabdomyosarcoma, and the extraskeletal variants of Ewing's and osteosarcoma. Chemotherapeutic complete remissions were not observed in patients with locally advanced disease, presumably secondary to the bulk of tumor involvement and the early assessment of response.

Twenty-five patients underwent surgical resection in an attempt to improve response. In all cases but one, surgery was performed in an attempt to create a complete remission. In the final case, the procedure was performed simply to decrease tumor bulk. Surgical resection resulted in complete remission in 15 patients, 60% of those operated on, and 30% of the total group (Table 3). In nine patients, minimal residual disease after surgery left them in good partial remission status. Overall, 22 of the 50 patients or 44% achieved complete remission either with chemotherapy or chemotherapy plus surgery. Fifteen patients or 30% had partial remission for an overall complete plus partial remission rate of 74%.

Time to progression from initiation of chemotherapy and survival were calculated for all patients (Fig. 1), and for subgroups of patients by response, and by type of disease – locally advanced versus metastatic. There was no significant difference by disease type; therefore, all patients were combined for assessment

Table 2. Continuous infusion CyADIC: Chemotherapy response of soft tissue sarcomas.

Sarcoma	Number of patients	Number of responses				
		Complete	Partial	Minor	Stable	Progression
MFH	13	1	6	0	1	5
Neurogenic	6	1	1	1	1	2
Angio	5	2	1	1	0	1
Leiomyo	5	0	3	0	1	1
Unclassified	5	0	2	1	2	0
Epithelioid	3	0	1	0	1	1
Synovial	2	0	2	0	0	0
Ewings	1	1	0	0	0	0
Osteo	1	1	0	0	0	0
Rhabdo	1	1	0	0	0	0
Other	8	0	4	1	3	0
Total	50	7 14%)	20 (40%)	4	9	10
		54%				

Table 3. Continuous infusion CyADIC: Effect of planned surgery.

	Number of patients	Final response	
		Complete	Partial
Surgery	25	15	9
No surgery	25	7	6
Total	50	22 (44%)	15 (30%)

of the effects of response on remission duration and survival. As in our previous studies, there were no significant differences between patients with chemotherapy-induced complete remission and those who achieved complete remission with the aid of surgery. Median time to progression for the entire group was 10 months and median survival 21 months. These figures are superior to those on our previous studies; however, they reflect primarily the improved rate of complete response obtained with combined chemotherapy and surgery. For patients with partial remission, median time to progression was 9 months, and median survival 13 months. For patients with complete remission, median time to progression is 25 months and median survival has not yet been reached with 75% of patients surviving at 22 months. Although these results are encouraging,

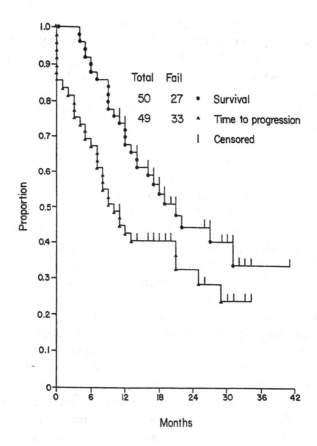

Fig. 1. Time to progression and survival all soft tissue sarcomas.

further observation and additional patient accrual will be necessary to determine whether the prolonged use of adriamycin has resulted in an increased proportion of patients who are cured or prolongation of the remission duration of those who are not.

The toxicity of the regimen is as might be expected from the same drugs given by the standard rapid-infusion schedule. Nausea and vomiting occurred in almost all patients, particularly on the first day of chemotherapy. Qualitatively, however, the degree of gastrointestinal disturbance was generally less than that seen with rapid infusion of the same drugs. Myelosuppression was significant, but was built into the protocol by the dosage escalation schema. Despite severe myelosuppression, however, only 21% of courses were associated with febrile neutropenic episodes, there were few documented infections, and no fatalities. Febrile neutropenic episodes occurred in 33% of the courses escalated to the third dose level. The most bothersome side effect was mucositis which was increased over that seen with single-dose administration of adriamycin. Overal 25% of courses were complicated by mucositis; however, mucositis became the dose limiting toxixity at the third dose level, affecting 58% of courses. At the doses used in this study, the continuous-infusion schedule did not diminish the frequency or severity of alopecia although the onset of total alopecia may have been somewhat delayed. Clinically significant cardiac toxicity was not observed.

Discussion and Conclusions

The use of a continuous-infusion chemotherapy program for patients with soft-tissue sarcomas in a combined modality approach utilizing surgery to remove residual disease whenever possible has resulted in our best overall result to date in regard to the incidence of complete remission, time to disease progression, and survival. Fourteen percent of patients achieved complete remission with chemo-therapy alone and 54% achieved complete or partial remission. These results are similar to those which we have obtained utilizing the standard CyVADIC regi-men with dose escalation. Since these results represent the effect of only three courses of chemotherapy in the majority of patients, it is possible that they might have been improved further had patients continued on the chemotherapy with-out surgery. Surgery, however, had a profound effect on the complete remission rate and ultimately the potential for cure by converting 30% of patients from lesser degrees of response to complete remission. Whether the prolonged admin-istration of adriamycin will indeed lead to longer remission duration and sur-vival and increased chance of cure remains a question. Preliminary data in this regard are encouraging, but more patients and longer follow-up will be needed to determine if this is indeed the case. In the meantime, we feel quite confident in recommending the regimen for general use since at the first two dose levels, it is generally better tolerated by patients than the standard CyADIC regimen at the same doses, particularly in terms of decreased intensity of nausea and vomiting. This and parallel studies have demonstrated that patients can be treated up to a cumulative adriamycin dose of 800 mg/m^2 using this schedule with careful, noninvasive cardiac monitoring. Although patients on this study have received over 1500 mg/m^2 of adriamycin, higher doses are not recommended routinely without the additional use of endomyocardial biopsies together with the non-invasive studies.

References

1. Gottlieb JA, Baker LH, Quagliana JM, Luce JK, Whitecar JP, Jr, Sinkovics JG, Rivkin SE, Brownlee R, Frei E, III: Chemotherapy of sarcomas with a combination of adriamycin and

dimethyl triazeno imidazole carboxamide. Cancer 30:1632–1638, 1972.

2. Gottlieb JA, Benjamin RS, Baker LH, O'Bryan RM, Sinkovics JG, Hoogstraten B, Quagliana JM, Rivkin SE, Bodey GP, Rodriquez V, Blumenschein GR, Saiki JH, Coltman C, Jr., Burgess MA, Sullivan P, Thigpen T, Bottomley R, Balcerzak S, Moon RE: Role of DTIC in the chemotherapy of sarcomas. Cancer Treat Rep 60:199–203, 1976.

3. Gottlieb JA, Baker LH, O'Bryan RM, Sinkovics JG, Hoogstraten B, Quagliana JM, Rivkin SE, Bodey GP, Rodriquez VT, Blumenschein GR, Saiki JH, Coltman C, Jr, Burgess MA, Sullivan P, Thigpen T, Bottomley R, Balcerzak S, Moon TE: Adriamycin used alone and in combination for soft tissue and bony sarcomas. Cancer Chemother Rep 6:271–282, 1975.

4. Benjamin RS, Baker LH, Rodriguez V, Moon TE, O'Bryan RM, Stephens RL, Sinkovics JG, Thigpen T, King GW, Bottomley R, Groppe CW, Jr, Bodey GP, Gottlieb JA: The chemotherapy of soft tissue sarcomas in adults. In: Management of Primary Bone and Soft Tissue Thors. Chicago: Year Book Medical Publisher, 1977, pp 309–315.

5. Yap BS, Baker LH, Sinkovics JG, Rivkin SE, Bottomley R, Thigpen T, Burgess MA, Benjamin RS, Bodey GP: Cyclophosphamide, Vincristine, Adriamycin, and DTIC combination chemotherapy for the treatment of advanced sarcomas. Cancer Treat Rep 64:93–98, 1980.

6. Yap BS, Rasmussen SL, Burgess MA, Sinkovics JG, Benjamin RS, Bodey GP: Prognostic factors in adults with advanced soft tissue sarcomas. Proc Am Soc Clin Oncol 21:473, 1980.

7. Yap BS, Sinkovics JG, Benjamin RS, Bodey GP: Survival and relapse patterns of complete responders in adults with advanced soft tissue sarcomas. Proc Am Soc Clin Oncol 20:352, 1979.

8. Legha SS, Benjamin RS, Mackay B, Ewer M, Wallace S, Valdivieso M, Rasmussen SL, Blumenschein GR, Freireich EJ: Reduction of doxorubicin cardiotoxicity by prolonged continuous intravenous infusion. Ann Inter Med 96:133–139, 1982.

9. Role of Radiotherapy

ROBERT D. LINDBERG

The role of radiation therapy in the treatment of adult soft tissue sarcomas has undergone a transition during the past two decades. Until recently, radical surgical excision has been considered the only curative treatment since soft tissue sarcomas were known to be 'radioresistant.' This concept of radioresistance was based on early published reports. In 1928, Rostock [1] reported on a collected series of 505 patients with soft tissue sarcoma. Although 78% of the sarcomas responded favorable immediately following irradiation, only 2.9% of the patients were cured as compared to a 30%, 5-year cure rate in another group of 550 patients treated by surgery alone. Thus, the concept of 'radioresistance' was firmly established and surgery became the treatment of choice.

Over the ensuing years, there has been considerable debate about the radiosensitivity of soft tissue sarcomas. Leucutia [2] observed that sarcomas had a widely divergent radiosensitivity as compared to other groups of tumors. Included in that sarcoma group, however, were the lymphosarcoma, osteosarcoma, and soft tissue sarcoma, which accounts for much of the confusion. One of the earliest publications showing the value of combined surgery and radiotherapy in the treatment of soft tissue sarcomas was by Leucutia in 1935 [2]. He reported a 34%, 5- to 12-year survival rate in a group of 101 patients. The rationale for combined surgery and radiotherapy was expressed by Leucutia [3] in 1950:

Whereas it would seem that in radioresistant types of sarcoma, as for example, the fibrosarcoma, neurogenic sarcoma, leiomyosarcoma, and rhabdomyosarcoma, irradiation in any form is out of place, practical experience shows that when it is used postoperatively, there is a definite improvement in the final results over those obtained by surgery alone. Recurrences are often observed less frequently, and the rate of 5 year survival is increased. The explanation of this lies in the fact that by irradiating the tumor bed and a wide surrounding area, the potential sources of new tumor foci, and perhaps, also the tumor cells left behind, are being destroyed through the secondary effect on normal tissue.

Baker, L.H. (ed.), Soft Tissue Sarcomas. ISBN 0-89838-584-9
© *1983 Martinus Nijhoff Publishers, Boston/The Hague/Dordrecht/Lancaster. Printed in the Netherlands.*

In the early 1950's Cade [4] reported the results of 128 patients with soft tissue sarcomas who were treated by three different methods. The cure rate for radiation therapy alone was 38.5% (10/26), for amputation 27.3% (6/22), and for wide excision and irradiation 61.3% (49/80). With the advent of megavoltage radiotherapy in the mid-1950s there was renewed interest in the treatment of soft tissue sarcomas by radiation therapy, either alone or in combination with surgery. In spite of the recent reports in the literature, considerable debate continues regarding the usefulness of radiation therapy. The concept of surgery alone as the curative approach for localized soft tissue sarcomas in adults persists to the present day [5].

There are three basic treatment approaches: (1) radiotherapy alone, (2) combined surgery and radiotherapy in which the radiotherapy may be given preoperatively or postoperatively, and (3) the use of chemotherapy as an adjuvant either to radiotherapy alone or combined with surgery.

Radiotherapy Alone

During the past 10 to 15 years, there have been few publications reporting the treatment of soft tissue sarcomas by radiation therapy alone. In 1968, McNeer *et al.* [6] reported a 5-year determinate survival rate of 56% (14/25) for patients with sarcomas treated by radiation therapy. In contrast, in 1973, The University of Texas M.D. Anderson Hospital (MDAH) [7] reported on 35 patients treated with high-dose irradiation (7000–7500 cGy-rad) using conventional fractionation techniques. The two-year disease-free survival rate was only 17.1% (6/35); three of the six survivors had local recurrences and were salvaged by further surgery. The overall local recurrence rate was 65.7% (23/35). Reitan and Kaalhus [8] demonstrated that only 2 of 15 patients with liposarcomas treated by radiotherapy alone had complete regressions lasting more than one year. Recently, Salinas *et al.* [9] reported encouraging results with fast neutron therapy in 29 patients with locally advanced lesions. These tumors ranged from 8 to 22 cm in diameter. They reported local control in 69% (20/29) with 5 to 62 month follow-up.

There have been reports in the literature [6, 10] indicating that certain soft tissue sarcomas, especially liposarcoma, are more radiosensitive and thus more radiocurable than other types of sarcoma. Recently, the American Joint Committee [11] proposed a staging system incorporating the grade of the lesion. Using the prognostic criteria of grade, size, and location of lesion, there are no published reports which show that one histological subtype of sarcoma is more radiocurable than others.

In general, there is little enthusiasm for the treatment of localized soft tissue sarcomas by radiation therapy alone for cure using conventional modalities and techniques. Patients with unresectable lesions or those having contraindications to surgery will benefit from conventional radiation therapy, but this is usually considered palliative.

Combined Surgery and Radiotherapy

Recent surgical reports [12, 13] have shown that more than 50% of patients with localized soft tissue sarcomas arising in the extremities require amputation or disarticulation to obtain adequate surgical margins. The combination of a more conservative surgical procedure and radiation therapy is an attempt to preserve a functional limb. Two of the major parameters that predict the radiocurability of any malignant tumor are: (1) the volume of the tumor (the number of tumor cells), and (2) the percentage of severely hypoxic cells in the tumor. The rationale for combined treatment is that surgery removes the large, bulky, gross tumor with hypoxic radioresistant cells, and radiation therapy destroys the subclinical sarcoma cells beyond the periphery of the surgical excision. This concept has been shown to be effective in carcinomas of the head and neck [14] and breast [15] i.e., 5000 cGy (rad) tumor dose in five weeks, sterilizes more than 90% of the subclinical disease. This concept is even more applicable to soft tissue sarcomas since most of the soft tissue sarcomas are significantly larger with a greater number of tumor cells.

The radiation therapy may be given either before or after surgery. The arguments about preoperative versus postoperative radiation therapy enumerated for other malignant tumors also apply to soft tissue sarcomas.

Postoperative Radiation Therapy

Recently there have been a number of reports [6, 16, 17] demonstrating the value of postoperative radiation therapy. McNeer *et al.* [6] reported a 69% 5 year survival rate in 98 patients treated by surgery and postoperative radiotherapy.

At MDAH the majority of patients are seen after an excisional biopsy or a 'shelling-out.' These patients must be critically evaluated in order to assure that all gross tumor had been removed. A conservative re-excision of the local area is necessary: (1) if there is known gross residual tumor, (2) when the gross tumor was removed in fragments, and (3) when there is a high probability of gross residual tumor. Patients presenting with operable gross tumors, either untreated or recurrent, undergo re-excision with a limited margin of normal tissue.

Radiation therapy is usually started within three to four weeks post-operatively when healing is complete. The radiotherapy techniques vary with the location, size, and grade of the primary tumor. The surgical field is irradiated with a generous margin using a shrinking field technique after 5000 cGy (rad) tumor dose. Currently the total dose is 6000 cGy in six weeks for low grade lesions, and 6500 cGy in 6–1/2 weeks for intermediate and high grade lesions. The details of the radiotherapy techniques have been published previously [18, 19].

In 1981, MDAH [16] published the results of 300 patients with localized soft tissue sarcomas treated by conservative surgery and postoperative radiation therapy. The lesions were classified according to the American Joint Committee Staging System. The two-year disease-free survival rate was 74% (222/300), for all patients and 78.5% (157/200) for patients with extremity lesions. The five-year absolute disease-free survival rates were 61.3% (103/168), and 69.4% (75/108) respectively (Table 1). The combination of conservation surgery and postoperative radiation therapy conserved a functional limb in 84.5% (169/200) of the patients with extremity lesions. The incidence of local failure, rate of distant metastases, and the determinate survival rate was also reported according to the American Joint Committee Staging System (Table 2) which demonstrates the prognostic value of the system.

Coe *et al.* [17] reported the recent experience for the Stanford Cade Department in London. The local control rate with excision and postoperative radiotherapy was 92% (46/50), the 2- and 5-year actuarial survival rate being 88% and 66% respectively.

In 1975, the National Cancer Institute started a prospective randomized trial comparing the effectiveness of amputation versus limited resection with postoperative radiation therapy in patients with extremity lesions. The preliminary results [20] indicate that the local control is equal in both arms but the final results are not yet available.

Table 1. Conservation surgery and postoperative radiotherapy: Absolute survival – free of disease.

Site	2 year 1963–1977	5 year 1963–1974
Head and neck	69.2% (18/26)	63.2% (12/19)
Trunk – abdomen	61.9% (13/21)	33.3% (5/15)
– other	64.2% (34/53)	42.3% (11/26)
Upper extremity	82.5% (52/63)	73.7% (28/38)
Lower extremity	76.6% (105/137)	67.1% (47/70)
Total	74% (222/300)	61.3% (103/168)

Adapted with permission from *Cancer* 47:2391–2397, 1981.

Table 2. Conservation surgery and postoperative radiotherapy: Relapse and survival versus AJC stage trunk and extremities[a]

Stage	Local failure	Distant metastasis	Determinate[b] survival
I A	6.3% (2/32)	3.1% (1/32)	96.7% (29/30)
B	12.9% (4/31)	6.4% (2/31)	89.3% (25/28)
II A	10.4% (5/48)	16.7% (8/48)	83.3% (40/48)
B	30.7% (23/75)	36% (27/75)	58.1% (43/74)
III A	31.6% (6/19)	21.1 (4/19)	68.4% (13/19)
B	27.1% (13/48)	52.1% (25/48)	40.0% (18/45)
	20.9% (53/253)	26.5% (67/253)	68.9% (168/244)

[a] Abdominal lesions excluded.
[b] Eliminates four patients dead of second primary, and five patients dead of intercurrent disease.
Adapted with permission from *Cancer* 47:2391–2397, 1981.

Preoperative Radiation Therapy

In 1963, Atkinson *et al.* [21] reported on 15 patients who were treated by preoperative radiotherapy (4500 cGy-rad in four to five weeks) followed by surgery six weeks later. At a median 41-month follow-up there was one local failure and no distant metastasis.

At MDAH in 1971, a clinical study [22] was started in patients with massive soft tissue sarcomas in 1976. Due to the size and location of the primary lesion, these patients were not candidates for conservation surgery, but would have required an ablation i.e., amputation, disarticulation, or forequarter or hind-quarter resection. These patients received preoperative irradiation, 5000 cGy (rad) tumor dose in five weeks to 6000 cGy (rad) in six weeks. Four to six weeks late, a conservative excision is attempted. Only one of the first 50 patients required ablative surgery. This patient presented with a 23 cm malignant fibro-histiocytoma of the thigh. A hip disarticulation was required to remove the gross tumor. The pathology report showed no tumor in the 18 cm mass. Nineteen of the 50 patients were treated between 1971 and August 1976, and therefore have a minimum 5-year follow-up. The primary tumors ranged from 10 to 28 cm in diameter with an average diameter of 14.2 cm and a median diameter of 14 cm. Fourteen of the 19 patients (73.7%) are living free of disease (Table 3). One additional patient developed lung metastases at 53 months which was treated surgically. Although this patient is free of disease at 65 months, he is listed under 'distant metastases' in Table 3 since only 12 months have elapsed since surgery.

Table 3. Radiotherapy followed by surgery: 1971 to August 1976.

Locale	Number of patients	5 year NED	Local failure	Distant metastasis
Thigh	14	11[a]	0	3
Leg	2	1	0	1
Upper extremity	3	2	0	1[b]
Total	19	14	0	5

[a] One patient developed lung metastases at 2 months – treated by chemotherapy and radiotherapy – currently NED at 62 months.
[b] Patient developed lung metastases at 53 months – treated by surgery – currently NED at 65 months.

Three of the 19 patients had minor complications, i.e., wound slough at 2, 4, and 8 months after surgery. One patient had a major complication, a fractured femur at 82 months. Currently, this patient walks with a leg brace.

Suit *et al.* [23] reported on 36 patients receiving preoperative radiotherapy at Massachusetts General Hospital. Conservative resection was not performed on seven patients: (1) amputation was the planned procedure in three patients, (2) amputation was necessary in one patient because of lack of tumor regression, and (3) in three patients exploration showed that resection was not feasible because of tumor extension. Twenty-five of the 36 patients who had the planned surgery have been followed 1 to 8 years. There has been one local recurrence, and 10 patients have developed distant metastasis. Thus, 56% (14/25) are living free of disease.

Adjuvant Chemotherapy

In the early 1970s, an analysis of the MDAH patients showed that despite surgery and postoperative radiation therapy, intermediate- and high-grade sarcomas larger than 5 cm in diameter have a 33% incidence of local recurrence and a 52.4% incidence of distant metastases [24]. Because of the high incidence of local recurrence and distant metastasis, a randomized study was started in October 1973, using adjuvant chemotherapy in this subset of sarcoma patients. Patients were randomized to receive either: (1) surgery and postoperative radiation therapy, or (2) surgery and concomitant radiotherapy and chemotherapy consisting of vincristine, Adriamycin, and Cytoxan. Actinomycin-D was substituted for Adriamycin after dose levels reached 420 mg/m². The preliminary results [25] showed that in patients receiving chemotherapy, there was an unacceptable level of toxicity without improvement in the disease-free survival rate.

Table 4. Randomized study – VACAR[a]: October 1973 – August 1976. Follow-up: 48 to 83 months.[b]

Treatment	Adjuvant chemotherapy	Control group
Total patients	30	28
Local failure	3 (10%)	10 (36%)
Distant metastases	15 (50%)	10 (36%)
Disease free survival	14 (47%)	13 (46%)
Living – NED	14 (47%)	18 (64%)[c]

[a] Conservation surgery, postoperative radiotherapy with adjuvant chemotherapy (vincristine, adriamycin, cytoxan, and actinomycin-D).
[b] 2/58 patients have less than 60 months follow-up.
[c] 5/10 with local failure are NED with surgical salvage.

The current results with a 48 to 83 month follow-up show that the continuous disease-free survival rate is essentially the same in both groups of patients (Table 4). At the time of the last analysis, the disease-free survival rate was higher in patients who did not receive adjuvant chemotherapy (64% versus 47%) since five of the 10 local recurrences in the control group were salvaged by further surgery and are living free of disease.

In 1978, the Southwest Oncology Group opened a study to test the efficacy of adjuvant Adriamycin and DTIC in high-risk patients with localized soft tissue sarcomas treated by conservative surgery and postoperative irradiation therapy. The study was closed in 1980 due to lack of patient accession.

Recently, chemotherapy has been added to the armamentarium of limb salvage surgery with radiation therapy in the treatment of localized soft tissue sarcomas of the extremities. Stehlin *et al.* [26] reported the use of hyperthermia, perfusion using Melphalan and Actinomycin-D, preoperative irradiation (3000 cGy in three weeks), and local excision in 17 patients. Postoperative radiotherapy (an additional 3000 cGy in three weeks) was added if residual disease was found at the time of surgery. Local control was achieved in 88% (15/17) of the patients. In 1980, Eilber *et al.* [27] reported on 65 patients with extremity soft tissue sarcomas treated by intra-arterial Adriamycin, preoperative radiotherapy (3500 cGy in two weeks), and radical en bloc resection. With a median follow-up of 22 months, there have been only two local recurrences. Four patients, however, required primary amputation to obtain tumor clearance. The actuarial 5-year survival rate was 75%.

124

Summary

The role of radiotherapy in the treatment of adults with soft tissue sarcomas has changed. During the past 20 years, three important factors have influenced that change: (1) the widespread use of megavoltage radiation therapy, (2) the changing concept of the 'radiosensitivity' of soft tissue sarcomas, and (3) the concept of radiotherapy in the treatment of subclinical disease. Thus, radiotherapy is not a substitute for surgical excision, but rather a valuable adjuvant.

Radiation therapy has played a significant role in advancing the concept of limb-salvage procedures for extremity lesions. For small and moderate-sized lesions, the combination of conservation surgery and postoperative radiation therapy has achieved the same absolute 5-year disease free survival rate as radical surgery (69.4%), while maintaining a functional extremity in 85% of the patients.

Various approaches are being used for the treatment of extensive or massive sarcomas including preoperative irradiation, with or without chemotherapy, in an attempt to maintain a functional limb. Although the experience is limited, these conservative approaches appear to be justified. Thus, primary amputation as the initial treatment of extremity soft tissue sarcomas is very rarely necessary.

References

1. Rostock P: Indikationsstellung and dauerertoig der rontgenbestrahlung bei sarkomen. Fortschr d Therap 4:241, 1928.
2. Leucutia T: Radiotherapy of sarcoma of the soft parts. Radiology 25:403, 1935.
3. Leucutia T: Treatment of disease of the skeletal system, joints, and soft tissues. In: Clinical Therapeutic Radiology. New York: Thomas Nelson and Sons, 1950.
4. Cade S: Soft tissue tumors: Their natural history and treatment. Proc R Soc Med 44:19, 1951.
5. Fortner JG: Soft tissue sarcomas. Clin Bull 5:62, 1975.
6. McNeer GP, Cantin J, Chu F, Nickson JJ: Effectiveness of radiotherapy in the management of sarcoma of soft tissues. Cancer 22:391–397, 1968.
7. Lindberg RD: The role of radiation therapy in the treatment of soft tissue sarcoma in adults. In: Proceedings of Seventh National Cancer Conference. Philadelphia: JB Lippincott Co, 1973, p 883.
8. Reitan JB, Kaalhus O: Radiotherapy of liposarcomas. Br J Radiol 53:969–975, 1980.
9. Salinas R, Hussey DH, Fletcher GH, Lindberg RD, Martin RG, Peters LJ, Sinkovics JG: Experience with fast neutron therapy for locally advanced sarcomas. Int J Radiat Oncol Biol Phys 6:267–272, 1980.
10. del Regato JA: Radiotherapy of soft tissue sarcomas. JAMA 185:216–218, 1963.
11. Russell WO, Cohn J, Enzinger F, Hajdu SI, Heise H, Martin RG, Meissner W, Miller WT, Schmitz RL, Suit HD: A clinical and pathological staging system for soft tissue sarcomas. Cancer 40:1562–1570, 1977.
12. Simon MA, Enneking WF: The management of soft tissue sarcomas of the extremities. J Bone Joint Surg 58A(3):317–327, 1976.
13. Simon MA, Spanier SS, Enneking WF: Management of adult soft tissue sarcomas of the extremities. Ann Surg 11:363–402, 1979.

14. Fletcher GH: Elective irradiation of subclinical disease in cancers of the head and neck. Cancer 29:1450–1454, 1972.
15. Fletcher GH: Local results of irradiation in the primary management of localized breast cancer. Cancer 29:545–551, 1972.
16. Lindberg RD, Martin RG, Romsdahl MM, Barkley HT: Conservation surgery and postoperative radiotherapy in 300 adults with soft tissue sarcomas. Cancer 47:2391–2397, 1981.
17. Coe MA, Madden FJ, Mould RF: The role of radiotherapy in the treatment of soft tissue sarcomas: A retrospective study 1958–73. Clin Radiol 32:42–51, 1981.
18. Lindberg RD, Fletcher GH, Martin RG: The management of soft tissue sarcomas in adults: Surgery and postoperative radiotherapy. J Radiol Electrol 56:761–767, 1975.
19. Lindberg RD: Soft tissue sarcoma. In: Textbook of Radiotherapy, Fletcher GH (ed). Philadelphia: Lea & Febiger, 1980 (3rd ed.), pp 922–942.
20. Rosenberg SA, Kent H, Costa J, Webber BL, Young R, Chabner B, Baker AR, Brennan MF, Chretien PB, Cohen MH, deMoss EV, Sears HF, Scipp C, Simon R: Prospective randomized evaluation of the role of limb-sparing surgery, radiation therapy, and adjuvant chemoimmunotherapy in the treatment of adult soft tissue sarcomas. Surgery 84:62–69, 1978.
21. Atkinson L, Garvan JM, Newton NC: Behavior and management of soft connective tissue sarcomas. Cancer 16:1552–1562, 1963.
22. Martin RG, Lindberg RD, Russell WO: Preoperative radiotherapy and surgery in the management of soft tissue sarcoma. In: Management of Primary Bone and Soft Tissue Tumors. Chicago: Year Book Medical Publishers, 1977, pp 299–307.
23. Suit HD, Proppe KH, Monkin HJ, Wood WC: Preoperative radiation therapy for sarcoma of soft tissue. Cancer 47:2269–2274, 1981.
24. Lindberg RD: Unpublished data 1972.
25. Lindberg RD, Murphy WK, Benjamin RS, Sinkovics JG, Martin RG, Romsdahl MM, Jesse RH, Russell WO: Adjuvant chemotherapy in the treatment of primary soft tissue sarcomas: A preliminary report. In: Management of Primary Bone and Soft Tissue Tumors. Chicago: Year Book Medical Publishers, 1977, pp 343–352.
26. Stehlin JS, de Ipolyi PD, Giovanella BC, Gutierrez AE, Anderson RF: Soft tissue sarcomas of the extremity. Multidisciplinary therapy employing hyperthermia perfusion. Am J Surg 130:643–646, 1975.
27. Eiber FR, Mirra JJ, Grant TT, Wersenburger T, Morton DL: Is amputation necessary for sarcomas? A seven-year experience with limb salvage. Ann Surg 192:431–438, 1980.

10. Chemotherapy of Disseminated Soft Tissue Sarcomas

LAURENCE H. BAKER

In 1972, adriamycin was introduced into clinical trial and quickly became identified as the single most important drug for the management of disseminated sarcomas. Previously, there were scattered reports in the literature indicating that different sarcomas were responsive to chemotherapeutic drugs, principally cyclophosphamide, actinomycin, and vincristine. Relatively few of these series had sufficient numbers of patients treated in a similar therapeutic regime however. Review of this early data suggests that metastatic sarcomas rarely responded 20% of the time or more. Most of those remissions were quite incomplete and short lasting and thus, of relatively little clinical benefit to the patient. Table 1 [1–6] summarizes major experiences with adriamycin as a single therapy.This data suggests that adriamycin as a single agent produces response rates of approximately 25%. The second drug whose investigation actually predated the investigation of adriamycin reported by Gottlieb et al. was DTIC (Dimethyl Trianzeno Immidazole Carboxamide). In Gottlieb's phase II trial 17% of 53 patients treated had responded to the DTIC [7, 8].

Concurrent with these clinical efforts, important pre-clinical studies were also being undertaken in the early 1970's primarily at the National Cancer Institute, as well as at the Southern Research Institute. These studies suggest that adriamycin and DTIC [9] could be combined in near full doses with the efficacy of the combination at least additive and not associated with an increase in toxicity. Thus the life span of mice bearing L1210 leukemia treated with the combination was significantly longer than animals treated with either agent alone. Similar results were also seen in a number of solid tumor systems including B16 malignant melanoma and C3^H adenocarcinoma.

At the end of 1971, the Southwest Oncology Group began a broad phase II trial for metastastic sarcomas utilizing adriamycin 60 mg/m^2 on day 1 and DTIC at a dose of 250 mg/m^2 given intravenously on days 1 through 5. This trial accrued 234 patients of which 9% of these patients achieved a complete clinical response, and 26% a partial response. It was also noted that the median survival of responders was 14 months. Duration of survival in the responding patients to adriamycin alone was 8 months. From the initial combination therapy of ad-

Baker, L.H. (ed.), Soft Tissue Sarcomas. ISBN 0-89838-584-9

Table 1. Adriamycin in soft tissue sarcomas.

Schedule	CR	PR	Cases	%	References
60–70 mg/m^2 q 3 wk	2	13	49	31	O'Bryan [1]
60–90 mg/m^2 q 3 wk	0	44	130	34	Blum [2]
75 mg/m^2 infused 72 h					
20–25 mg/m^2/d × 3	0	2	15	13	Creagan [3]
q 3 wk					
0.4 mg/kg days 1, 23, 8, 9, 10	1	6	41	15	Cruz [4]
q 2wk					
70 mg/m^2 q 3 wk	3	8	39	28	Schoenfeld [5]
25 mg/m^2 vs. 50 mg/m^2 q 3 wk	1	22	82	28	O'Bryan [6]
45 mg/m^2 vs. 70 mg/m^2 q 3 wk					

riamycin and DTIC several prognostic factors were further identified. For example, even within leiomyosarcomas when the primary site was in the genitourinary of gynecological system there was a 53% response rate vs. 21% in patients in which the primary site was the gastrointestinal site. Sites of metastases were also important and as with most chemotherapy studies soft tissue lesions were found to respond more frequently than did the bony lesions. The worst response rate perhaps was the CNS due to poor penetration of these drugs into this system.

Sequential additions of vincristine and cyclophosphamide were then made to the adriamycin- DTIC regime [10, 11, 12]. The addition of vincristine (VANIC) did not improve response rates or survival. Cyclophosphamide known to be active in childhood sarcomas was added, resulting in the CY-VA-DIC combination. More than 600 patients have now been treated with this basic regime as is reported in the literature. Response rates have varied by author from 30 to 57%.

Only one adriamycin-DTIC combination has had a significantly lower response rate than 30% and that was the trial of Creagen *et al.* [13], in which they reported an 11% response rate of 54 patients treated with vincristine, adriamycin and DTIC. However in this trial patients were re-treated at 5 week intervals vs. the traditional 3 week schedule. The results of combination chemotherapy are summarized in Table 2 [4, 5, 9, 10, 11, 13–25].

There are relatively few randomized prospective trials comparing different therapy regimes in soft tissue sarcomas. Benjamin *et al.* [11] compared the combination of CY-VA-DIC vs. CY-VA-DAC (cytoxan, adriamycin, vincristine, and actinomycin-D). The trial suggested that the DTIC containing four drug combination was superior to the actinomycin-D containing four drug regime. The trial of Rosenbaum and co-workers compared adriamycin to the drug combinations of vincristine, actinomycin-D and cytoxan vs. cytoxan, vincristine, and adriamycin. In this trial, adriamycin was superior to the VAC

Table 2. Combinations.

Combinations	CR	PR	Evaluable	%	References
Actinomycin-D + vincristine + cyclophosphamide q 4 wk	2	1	59	5	Schoenfeld [5]
Actinomycin-D + vincristine + cyclophosphamide q 4 wk	1	7	17	47	Jacobs [14]
Actinomycin-D + vincristine + cyclophosphamide q 5 wk	1	4	61	8	Creagan [13]
Adriamycin + DTIC q 3 wk	25	67	218	42	Gottlieb [9]
Adriamycin + DTIC q 3 wk	11	14	79	32	Baker [15]
Adriamycin + DTIC q 3 wk (single dose)	1	5	18	33	Saiki [16]
Adriamycin + vincristine + DTIC q 3 wk	10	35	107	42	Gottlieb [17]
Adriamycin + vincristine + DTIC q 5 wk	1	5	54	11	Creagan [13]
Adriamycin + DTIC + vincristine + cyclophosphamide q 3 wk	21	42	125	50	Yap [18]
Adriamycin + DTIC + vincristine + cyclophosphamide q 3 wk	8	14	60	37	Pinedo [10]
Adriamycin + DTIC + vincristine + cyclophosphamide q 3 wk	27	80	229	45	Benjamin [11]
Adriamycin + DTIC + cyclophosphamide q 3 wk	12	21	95	35	Baker [15]
Adriamycin + DTIC + cyclophosphamide q 3 wk (continuous infusion)	4	8	21	57	Benjamin [11]
Adriamycin + DTIC + cyclophosphamide	4	9	23	45	Blum [19]
Adriamycin + vincristine + cyclophosphamide + actinomycin-D q 3 wk	25	55	224	36	Benjamin [11]
Adriamycin + DTIC + actinomycin-D q 3 wk	9	15	98	24	Baker [15]
Adriamycin + methyl-CCNU	3	17	41	49	Rivkin [20]
Adriamycin + methyl-CCNU vincristine	0	10	22	45	Shiv [21]
Adriamycin + streptozotocin	0	2	14	1	Chang [22]
Adriamycin + cytoxan + methotrexate	4	38	140	30	Lowenbraun [23]
Adriamycin + methotrexate (HD) + vincristine	1	2	14	2	Kaufman [24]

Table 2. (Continued)

Combinations	CR	PR	Evaluable	%	References
Adriamycin + methotrexate (HD) + vincristine + DTIC	0	2	5	4	Kaufman [24]
Adriamycin + cytoxan + vincristine	3	9	56	21	Schoenfeld [5]
Actinomycin D + L-Pam	0	1	25	4	Cruz [4]
Actinomycin D + L-Pam + vincristine	0	0	26	–	Cruz [4]
Actinomycin D + L-Pam + cycloleucine	0	0	25	–	Cruz [4]
Actinomycin D + chlorambucil	0	5	40	13	Golbey [25]
Actinomycin D + chlorambucil + methotrexate	0	8	40	20	Golbey [25]
Vincristine + methotrexate + adriamycin + actinomycin D (VMAD)	0	14	32	44	Shiv [21]
Vincristine + methotrexate + adriamycin + actinomycin-D (OMAD) + DTIC + chlorambucil (ALOMAD)	0	13	41	32	Shiv [21]
Vincristine + methotrexate + adriamycin + DTIC + cytoxan (CYVMAD)	0	7	29	24	Shiv [21]

regime (Table 3) [5]. A third comparative trial of Cruz and co-workers suggested the superiority of adriamycin alone in comparison to combinations of actino-mycin-D and phenylalanine mustard; actinomycin-D, phenylalanine mustard, and vincristine; and actinomycin-D, phenylalanine mustard and cycloleucine [4].

A recently completed trial of Baker *et al.* asked the question as to whether or not a third drug added to the adriamycin-DTIC combination would improve response and/or survival. In this trial adriamycin-DTIC and actinomycin-D respective overall response rates were 33%, 38%, and 22%. No difference could be seen in terms of the frequency of completed response (15%, 13%, and 8%). Median survival for the three therapy groups were 37 weeks, 45 weeks, and 50 weeks. It was concluded from that trial that neither Cytoxan nor actinomycin-D were of sufficient clinical benefit in addition to the adriamycin-DTIC combinations (Table 4).

The most important biological phenomenon in treating disseminated soft tissue sarcomas appears to be the clear cut dose response relationship in the use of adriamycin. Thus, some of the disparity in reported trials of adriamycin

Table 3. ECOG study 2374.

Treatment	Complete response	Partial response	Evaluable patients	% response
Adriamycin	4	10	50	28%
Adriamycin, vincristine, cyclophosphamide	3	9	56	21%
Actinomycin-D, vincristine, cyclophosphamide (VAC)	2	1	59	5%

Table 4.

	Adriamycin DTIC	Adriamycin DTIC Cyclophosphamide	Adriamycin DTIC Actinomycin-D
Doses: Adriamycin 60 mg/m² d 1 DTIC 250 mg/m² dl-5 Cytoxan 1000 mg/m² d 1 Actinomycin-D 1.5 mg/m² d 3			
Fully evaluable cases	73	92	86
Complete response %	15	13	8
Partial response %	18	25	14
Median survival (weeks)	37	45	50
Median duration of response (weeks)	26	30	23
Severe or worse toxicity (%)	58	68	64

combinations may be explained in part by the degree of mild suppression acceptable to the treating physician. For example, patients whose white counts are lower than 1000 cells/mm² do significantly better than patients who experience little if any mild suppression. In the most recent study of Baker *et al.*, response rates in patients who had a white count nadir at or above 3000 had an overall response rate of 21% in comparison to patients who were made myelosuppressed whose response rate was 56%. Another prognostic factor unexplained thus far seems to be the importance of the sex of the patient. In almost all studies reported, women tend to survive longer than men with similar disease. In this most recent study quoted above the median survival of women was 55 weeks vs. the 36 weeks for men.

Another important accomplishment of this recent study was analysis following mandatory pathology review for a panel of experts. Previously, little data was available regarding the chemosensitivity of the various histologic subtypes. This study suggests that the prognosis of rhabdomyosarcoma appears to be the poorest while that of leiomyosarcoma and liposarcoma being the best of the studied group. An intermediate prognosis is given to malignant fibrous histiocy-

132

Table 5. Response and survival of histologic subtypes.

	Number of patients	Complete response and partial response (%)	Median survival
Leiomyosarcoma	73	33	58
Malignant fibrohistiocytoma	43	21	32
Liposarcoma	16	19	69
Rhabdomyosarcoma	14	29	26
Neurogenic sarcoma	14	29	36
Hemangiosarcoma	12	25	34
Synovial sarcoma	10	30	30
Fibrosarcoma	7	57	41
Miscellaneous	34	41	31

toma and of neurosarcomas (Table 5).

Unfortunately, since the mid-70's little improvement has been accomplished in the treatment of patients with disseminated sarcomas. It appears that an adriamycin-based combination is currently the treatment of choice. Unfortunately, no new drug has been identified that can be added to the adriamycin-based therapy that has provided significant improvement. In the chapter on intravenous infusion, data is presented suggesting that adriamycin given as a continuous infusion enhances the duration of adriamycin administration which in some patients leads to prolonged complete or good partial response. Further it is suggested by Yap *et al.* [18] and Bejamin *et al.* [11], that surgical excision following partial remission of patients with disseminated sarcomas is essentially equivalent to complete remission obtained by drug therapy alone. This retrospective review and observation requires prospective confirmation.

It is also clear from all these studies that partial remission is not of major clinical importance. Partial responses are relatively brief and the toxicity from these combinations is brisk. Complete responses occurring between 10 and 15 percent of the time in the various series however do translate to clinically useful therapeutic regimes. Unfortunately, since the mid-70's little if any has been accomplished to improve upon the complete response rate.

References

1. O'Bryan RM, Luce JK, Talley RW *et al.*: Phase II evaluation of adriamycin in human neoplasia. Cancer 31:1–8, 1973.
2. Blum RH: An overview of studies with adriamycin (NSC-123127) in the United States. Cancer Chemother Rep 6:247–251, 1975.

3. Creagan ET, Hahn RG, Ahmann DL *et al.*: A clinical trial adriamycin (NSC 123127) in advanced sarcomas. Oncology 34:90–91, 1977.
4. Cruz AB Jr., Thames EA Jr., Aust. JB *et al.*: Combination chemotherapy for soft tissue sarcomas: A phase III study. J Surg Oncol 11: 313–323, 1979.
5. Schoenfeld DA, Rosenbaum C, Horton J, *et al.*: A comparison of adriamycin versus vincristine and adriamycin and cyclophosphamide versus vincristine, actinomycin-D, and cyclophosphamide for advanced sarcoma. Cancer 50:2757–2762, 1982.
6. O'Bryan RM, Baker LH, Gottlieb JE *et al.*: Dose response evaluation of adriamycin in human neoplasia. Cancer 39:1940–1948, 1977.
7. Gottlieb JA, Benjamin RA, Baker LH *et al.*: Role of DTIC (NSC-45338) in the chemotherapy of sarcomas. Cancer Treat Rep 60:199–203, 1976.
8. Luce JK, Thurman WG, Isaacs BL *et al.*: Clinical trials with the antitumor agent 5-(3,3-dimethyl-1-triazeno)imidazole-4-carboxamide (NSC-45388). Cancer Chemother Rep 54:119–124, 1970.
9. Gottlieb JA, Baker LH, Quagliana JM *et al.*: Chemotherapy of sarcomas with a combination of adriamycin and dimethyl-triazeno-imidazole-carboxamide. Cancer 30:1632–1638, 1972.
10. Pinedo HM, Vendrik CPJ, Bramwell VHC *et al.*: Re-evaluation of the CYVADIC regimen for metastatic soft tissue sarcoma. Proc AACR and ASCO (abstr) C-228, 1978.
11. Benjamin RS, Gottlieb JA, Baker LH *et al.*: CYVADIC versus CYVADACT – a randomized trial of cyclophosphamide (CY), vincristine (V), and adriamycin (A) plus either dacarbazine (DIC), or actinomycin-D (DACT) in metastatic sarcomas. Proc Am Assoc Cancer Res Am Soc Clin Oncol, 17:256, 1976.
12. Baker LH: Unpublished data.
13. Creagan ET, Hahn RG, Ahmann DL *et al.*: A comparative clinical trial evaluating the combination of adriamycin, DTIC, and vincristine, the combination of actinomycin-D, cyclophosphamide, and vincristine, and a single agent, methyl-CCNU, in advanced sarcomas. Cancer Treat Rep 60:1385–1386, 1976.
14. Patten BM: Human Embryology. New York: McGraw-Hill, 1968.
15. Baker LH: Unpublished data.
16. Saiki JH: Unpublished data.
17. Gottlieb JA, Baker LH, Burgess MA *et al.*: Sarcoma chemotherapy. In: Cancer Chemotherapy Fundamental Concepts and Recent Advances, 19th Annual Clinical Conference in Cancer, 1974, MD. Anderson Hospital. Chicago: Year Book Medical Publishers, 1975.
18. Yap B, Baker LH, Sinkovics JG *et al.*: Cyclophosphamide, vincristine, adriamycin, and DTIC (CYVADIC) combination chemotherapy for the treatment of advanced sarcomas. Cancer Treat Rep 64: 93–98, 1980.
19. Blum RH, Carson JM, Wilson RE *et al.*: Successful treatment of metastatic sarcomas with cyclophosphamide, adriamycin, and DTIC (CAD). Cancer 46: 1722–1726, 1980.
20. Rivkin SE, Gottlieb JA, Thigpen T *et al.*: Methyl CCNU and adriamycin for patients with metastatic sarcomas. A Southwest Oncology Group Study. Cancer 46:446–451, 1980.
21. Shiv MH, Magill GB, Hopfan S: Recent trends in treatment of soft tissue sarcomas – Appendix A.: In: Pathology of Soft Tumors, Hajdu SI (ed). Philadelphia: Lea & Febiger, 1979, pp 537–542.
22. Chang P, Wiernik PH: Combination chemotherapy with adriamycin and streptozotocin. Clin Pharmacol Ther 20:605–610, 1976.
23. Lowenbraun S, Moffitt S, Smalley R *et al.*: Combination chemotherapy with adriamycin, cyclophosphamide and methotrexate in metastatic sarcomas. ASCO (abstr) 18:286, 1977.
24. Kaufman JH, Catane R, Douglass HO Jr.: Combined adriamycin, vincristine, and methotrexate. NY State J Med, 742–743, 1977.
25. Golbey R, Li MC, Kaufman RF: Actinomycin in the treatment of soft part sarcomas. James Ewing Society Scientific Program (abstr), 1968.

11. Phase II New Drug Trials in Soft Tissue Sarcomas

MICHAEL K. SAMSON

Doxorubicin, since its introduction into clinical trials in 1972, remains the single most important drug in the management of disseminated soft tissue sarcomas. The response rate to doxorubicin varies from 13–34% [1–4]. Several clinical trials have established that a dose–response relationship exists and may account for the variable response data observed [5–8]. Studies employing various combinations of doxorubicin including doxorubicin-DTIC, doxorubicin-DTIC-cyclophosphamide, doxorubicin-DTIC-actinomycin D, and doxorubicin-DTIC-cyclophosphamide-vincristine, have not been able to show any clear-cut superiority of a particular combination in terms of response rate, response duration or overall survival. In general, median response duration is around 6 months with survival approaching 2 years. Since the complete response rate to doxorubicin alone or in combination rarely exceeds 10%, with only an occasional patient having prolonged meaningful survival, efforts have continued to identify new drugs with activity against soft tissue sarcomas. Table 1 summarizes the various new drugs that have had a sufficient clinical trial in the treatment of patients with soft tissue sarcomas and the results of such studies.

From this review of phase II chemotherapeutic agents in soft tissue sarcomas, it is readily apparent that except for a few, no drug emerges from any study as clearly an active agent, deserving of being advanced to doxorubin-containing combinations. Notable exceptions may include high-dose (100–120 mg/m^2) cis-DDP and vindesine. Most of these trials include patients with at least one prior trial of chemotherapy, far advanced disease and poor performance status. For patients with solid tumors, these factors have significant impact on the likelihood of a response to any therapeutic modality. It is clear from experience with doxorubicin-containing combinations, a response rate of 30–50% is to be expected depending upon the aggressiveness of treatment and the acceptance of myelotoxicity. However, until the complete response rate approaches 50%, the impact on survival remains unsatisfactory. Clearly new, active agents are urgently needed. As newer agents with potential antitumor activity are identified, via the human tumor stem-cell assay system [38], human tumor xenografts, phase I clinical trials, or other mechanisms, new treatment strategies need to be implemented.

Baker, L.H. (ed.), Soft Tissue Sarcomas. ISBN 0-89838-584-9

© 1983 Martinus Nijhoff Publishers, Boston/The Hague/Dordrecht/Lancaster. Printed in the Netherlands.

Table 1. Phase II investigational drug trials in soft tissue sarcomas.

Drug	No. of eligible patients	No. of responses (%)	References
AMSA	23	1 (4)	Sordillo [9]
Anguidine	22	0 (0)	Thigpen [10]
Azotomycin	13	1 (8)	Chang [11]
	16	4 (25)	Weiss [12]
Baker's Antifol	25	0 (0)	Thigpen [13]
Carminomycin	48	13 (27)	Perevodchikova [14]
Chlorozotocin	27	0 (0)	Sordillo [15]
	21	0 (0)	Mouridsen [16]
	25	4 (16)	Talley [17]
Cycloleucine	11	0 (0)	Baker [18]
	98	6 (6)	Savlov [19]
Cytembena	10	0 (0)	Baker [20]
DDMP	15	1 (7)	Alberto [21]
cis-DDP	13	3 (23)	Karakousis [22]
	42	3 (7)	Samson [23]
	17	0 (0)	Bramwell [24]
Dianhydrogalactitol	27	0 (0)	Thigpen [25]
Dibromodulcitol	33	0 (0)	ECOG [26]
Diglycoaldehyde	20	0 (0)	Vosika [27]
Gallium nitrate	16	0 (0)	Samson [28]
Hexamethylmelamine	37	3 (8)	Borden [29]
ICRF 159	29	1 (3)	ECOG [30]
Methyl CCNU	15	0 (0)	Creagan [31]
	70	5 (7)	Tranum [32]
Piperazinedione	19	1 (5)	La Gasse [33]
Pyrazofurin	21	0 (0)	Cormier [34]
	24	0 (0)	Gralla [35]
Vindesine	46	3 (7)	Sordillo [36]
VM-26	17	0 (0)	Bleyer [37]

One proposal is that future phase II drug trials be limited to patients that have received only one previous chemotherapy trial and have a minimum performance status of 1 (Karnofsky 70–80). Another more controversial approach that merits serious consideration is the following: drug X, identified as a potential

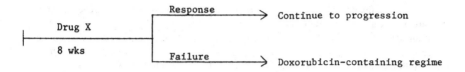

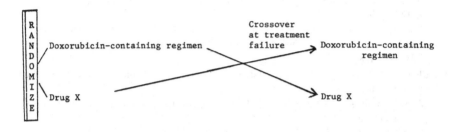

active agent via one of the aforementioned mechanisms, would be administered 'up front' to previously untreated patients for a stated treatment period, i.e. 8 weeks. At the completion of that time period those patients failing to respond would receive a doxorubicin-containing combination. If the patient were to respond (either CR or PR) it would be continued until disease progression were noted (Fig. 1). An alternate treatment strategy would be to randomize patients between drug X and a doxorubicin-containing combination, with provision for cross-over at that time in which progressive disease was noted (Fig. 2).

More work is needed on the basic biology of soft-tissue sarcomas, including the mechanisms of adriamycin sensitivity and resistance in addition to the vigorous pursuit of effective antitumor modalities. Both of these approaches are not mutually exclusive.

References

1. O'Bryan RM, Luce JK, Talley RW, Gottlieb JA, Baker LH, Bonadonna G: Phase II evaluation of adriamycin in human neoplasia. Cancer 32:1–8, 1973.
2. Blum RH: An overview of studies with adriamycin (NSC-123127) in the United States. Cancer Chemother Rep 6:247–251, 1975.
3. Creagan ET, Hahn RG, Ahmann DL, Bisel HF: A clinical trial of adriamycin (NSC-123127) in advanced sarcomas. Oncology 34:90–91, 1977.
4. Rosenbaum C, Schoenfeld D: Treatment of advanced tissue sarcoma. Proc ASCO & AACR 18:287, 1977.
5. O'Bryan RM, Baker LH, Gottliev JA, Rivkin S et al.: Dose response evaluation of adriamycin in human neoplasia. Cancer 39:1940–1948, 1977.

138

6. Gottlieb JA, Benjamin RS, Baker LH, O'Bryan RM *et al.*: Role of DTIC in the chemotherapy of sarcomas. Cancer Treat Rep 60:199–203, 1976.

7. Blum RH, Corson JM, Wilson RE, Greenberger JS *et al.*: Successful treatment of metastatic sarcomas with cyclophosphamide, adriamycin, and DTIC (CAD). Cancer 46:1722–1726, 1980.

8. Yap B, Baker LH, Sinkovics JC, Rivkin SE *et al.*: Cyclophosphamide, vincristine, adriamycin, and DTIC (CYVADIC) combination chemotherapy for the treatment of advanced sarcomas. Cancer Treat Rep 64:93–98, 1980.

9. Sordillo PP, Magill GB, Gralla RJ, Golby RB: Phase II evaluation of 4'-(9-Acridinylamino)-methanesulfon-in-anisidine (AMSA) in patients with advanced sarcoma. Cancer Treat Rep 64:1129–1130, 1980.

10. Thigpen JT, Vaughn C, Stuckey WJ: Phase trial of anguidine in patients with sarcomas unresponsive to prior chemotherapy: A Southwest Oncology Group Study. Cancer Treat Rep 65:881–882, 1981.

11. Chang P, Wiernik PH: Phase II study of azotomycin in sarcomas. Cancer Treat Rep 61:1719–1920, 1977.

12. Weiss AJ, Ramierez G, Grage T *et al.*: Phase II study of azotomycin (NSC-56654). Cancer Chemother Rep 52:611–614, 1968.

13. Thigpen JT, O'Bryan RM, Benjamin RS, Coltman CA Jr.: Phase II trial of Baker's antifol in metastatic sarcoma. Cancer Treat Rep 61:1485–1487, 1977.

14. Perevodchikova NI, Lichinitser MR, Gorfunova VA: Phase I clinical study of carminomycin: Its activity against soft tissue sarcomas. Cancer Treat Rep 61:1705–1707, 1977.

15. Sordillo PP, Magill GB, Gralla RJ: Chlorozotocin: Phase II evaluation in patients with advanced sarcomas. Cancer Treat Rep 65:513–514, 1981.

16. Mouridsen HT, Bramwell VHC, Lacave J, Metz R, Vendrik C, Hild J, McCreanney J, Sylvester R: A Phase II trial of the EORTC Soft Tissue and Bone Sarcoma Group. Cancer Treat Rep 65:509–511, 1981.

17. Talley RW, Samson MK, Brownlee RW, Samhouri AM, Fraile RJ, Baker LH: Phase II evaluation of chlorozotocin (NSC-178248) in advanced human cancer. Eur J Cancer 17:337–343, 1981.

18. Baker LH, Fraile RJ, Samson MK, Cummings GD: Phase II evaluation of cycloleucine in the treatment of patients with disseminated sarcomas. Cancer Treat Rep 65:358–359, 1981.

19. Savlov ED, MacIntyre JM, Knight E, Walter J: Comparison of doxorubicin and cycloleucine in the treatment of sarcomas. Cancer Treat Rep 65:21–27, 1981.

20. Baker LH, Samson MK, Izbicki RM: Phase I and II evaluation of cytembena in disseminated epithelial ovarian cancers and sarcomas. Cancer Treat Rep 60(9):1389–1391, 1976.

21. Alberto P, De Jager RL, Brugarolas A, Hansen HH, Cavalli F, Host H: Phase II study of diamino-dichlorophenyl-methylpyrimidine (DDMP) with folinic acid (CF) protection and rescue. Proc AACR & ASCO 20:323, 1979.

22. Karakousis CP, Holtermann OA, Holyoke ED: Cis-dichlorodiammineplatinum (II) in metastatic soft tissue sarcomas. Cancer Treat Rep 63:2071–2075.

23. Samson MK, Baker LH, Benjamin RS, Lane M, Plager C: Cis-dichlorodiammineplatinum (II) in advanced soft tissue and bony sarcomas: A Southwest Oncology Group Study. Cancer Treat Rep 63:2027–2029, 1979.

24. Bramwell VHC, Brugarolas A, Mouridsen HT, Cheix F, De Jager R, Van Oosterom AT, Vendrik CP, Pinedo HM, Sylvester R, De Pauw M: E.O.R.T.C. Phase II study of cisplatin in cyvadic-resistant soft tissue sarcoma. Eur J Cancer 15:1511–1513, 1979.

25. Thigpen JT, Samson MK: Phase II trial of dianhydrogalactitol in advanced soft tissue and bony sarcomas: A Southwest Oncology Group Study. Cancer Treat Rep 63:553–555, 1979.

26. Eastern Cooperative Oncology Group: Unpublished data.

27. Vosika GJ, Briscoe K, Carey RW, O'Connell JF, Perry MC, Budman D, Richards F III,

Coleman M: Phase II study of diglycoaldehyde in malignant melanomas and soft tissue sarcomas. Cancer Treat Rep 65:823–825, 1981.

28. Samson MK, Fraile RJ, Baker LH, O'Bryan R: Phase I-II trial of gallium nitrate (NSC-15200). Cancer Clin Trials 3:131–136, 1980.

29. Borden EC, Larson P, Ansfield FJ et al.: Hexamethylmelamine treatment of sarcomas and lymphomas. Med Pediatr Oncol 3:401–406, 1977.

30. Eastern Cooperative Oncology Group: Unpublished data.

31. Creagan ET, Hahn RG, Ahmann DL, Edmondson JH, Bisel HF, Eagan RT: A comparative clinical trial evaluating the combination of adriamycin, DTIC and vincristine, the combination of actinomycin D, cyclophosphamide and vincristine, and a single agent, methyl-CCNU in advanced sarcomas. Cancer Treat Rep 60:1385–1387, 1976.

32. Tranum BL, Haut A, Rivkin S, Weber E et al.: A Phase II study of methyl CCNU in the treatment of solid tumors and lymphomas: A Southwest Oncology Group Study. Cancer 35:1148–1153, 1975.

33. La Gasse L, Thigpen T, Morrison F: Phase II trial of piperazinedione in the treatment of advanced endometrial carcinoma, uterine sarcoma and vulvar carcinoma. Proc Am Assoc Cancer Res 20:388, 1979.

34. Cormier WJ, Hahn RG, Edmonson JH, Eagan RT: Phase II study in advanced sarcoma: Randomized trial of pyrazofurin versus combination cyclophosphamide, doxorubicin, and cis-dichlorodiammeplatinum (II) (CAP). Cancer Treat Rep 64:655–658, 1980.

35. Gralla RJ, Sordillo PP, Magill GB: Phase II evaluation of pyrazofurin in patients with metastatic sarcoma. Cancer Treat Rep 62:1573–1574, 1978.

36. Sordillo PP, Magill GB, Gralla RJ: Phase II evaluation of vindesine sulfate in patients with advanced sarcoma. Cancer Treat Rep 65:515–516, 1981.

37. Bleyer WA, Chard RL, Krivit W, Hammond D: Epipodophyllotoxic therapy of childhood neoplasia: A comparative phase II analysis of VM-26 and VP16-213. Proc AACR & ASCO 19:373, 1978.

38. Salmon SE, Meyskens F Jr., Alberts DS, Soehnlen B, Young L: New drugs in ovarian cancer and malignant melanoma: In vitro phase II screening with the human tumor stem cell assay. Cancer Treat Rep 65:1–12, 1981.

Index

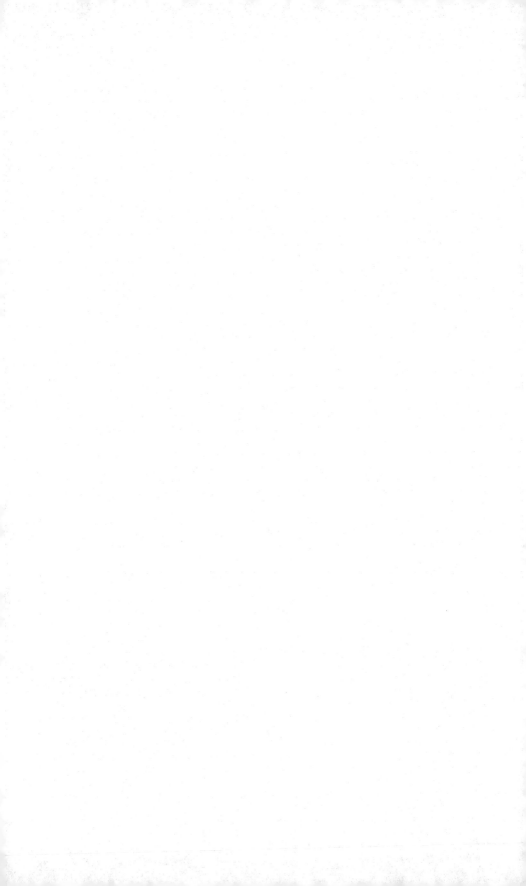